VICKY PHELAN

with Naomi Linehan

Overcoming

A Memoir

HACHETTE
BOOKS
IRELAND

First published in Ireland in 2019 by Hachette Books Ireland

Cataloguing in Publication Data is available from the British Library

ISBN 978 1 52931 870 8

Typeset in Sabon by redrattledesign.com

Printed and bound in Great Britain by Clays Ltd, Elcograf S.p.A.

The author and publishers would like to thank the following: Gwen Malone
Stenography Services, for permission to reproduce court transcripts in the
book; The Stunning, for permission to reproduce lyrics from 'This Happy
Girl'; the Pellenz family, the Murphy family, Paul Maxwell Photography, Joe
Cashin, Brian Lawless/PA Images, Collins Agency, True Media Photography
and Ann Power, for permission to reproduce images.

Hachette Books Ireland policy is to use papers that are natural, renewable
and recyclable products and made from wood grown in sustainable forests.
The logging and manufacturing processes are expected to conform to the
environmental regulations of the country of origin.

Hachette Books Ireland
8 Castlecourt Centre
Castleknock
Dublin 15, Ireland

A division of Hachette UK Ltd
Carmelite House, 50 Victoria Embankment, EC4Y 0DZ

www.hachettebooksireland.ie

Overcoming

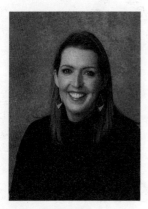

Vicky Phelan is mother to Amelia and Darragh, married to Jim and living in Limerick, Ireland. She is a lifelong learner and has always worked in the education field. She credits her education with giving her the tools to take on her greatest challenge – fighting for her life. She is a founding member of the 221+ CervicalCheck Patient Support Group and a powerful advocate for those affected. *Overcoming* is her first book.

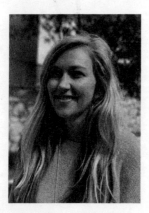

Naomi Linehan is an author, journalist and documentary-maker. She was born in Dublin and grew up in Zambia. *Overcoming* is her second book. Her first book, *Nowhere's Child*, was published by Hachette in 2015. It soon became a number one bestseller and has since been published internationally and has been translated into three different languages. Naomi worked for many years in radio in flagship current affairs and features programmes on Newstalk. She has also written for *The Irish Times* and has worked in the areas of international development and social entrepreneurship. She is currently producing a television documentary series soon to be aired on RTÉ.

For Amelia and Darragh, you are my reason for living.
It has all been for you.

1

A Horse Of A Different Colour

CANCER IS ALL ABOUT TREATMENT. One treatment after another, or sometimes several all at once. And each treatment leaves behind a layer of pain which, over time, turns you into a kind of scarecrow.

Not from the outside.

From the outside you might look fine; people even tell you you're looking great. But from the inside looking out, you're a ragged thing, a collection of old scars and new symptoms, a comically monstrous version of your old self.

They keep piling on the treatment for as long as you can physically stand it, until you keel over from the sheer weight of it all, and drop where you stand. Then they stop. After they've done 'everything we can'.

I know luck is a major player in all of this, but it wasn't the cancer in my body that turned me into a scarecrow, it was the cancer in the system. And that knowledge makes me angry. Well, let me tell you: they don't like you when you're angry. It scares the living daylights out of them.

It's hard to know where to start. 'Start at the beginning,' you might say.

But every chapter of your life has its own beginning.

I suppose I could start on the day I found out I was a scarecrow. But when I think back, something else keeps rising in my mind. Something oddly comical, that happened many years ago.

It keeps coming back to me, this memory. I don't exactly know why.

I'm out walking. My head is in a dark place. All of a sudden, out of nowhere, a black horse appears. I hear him before I see him, the noise of his hooves against the concrete.

Coming right for me, gathering speed.

I'm running as fast as I can.

A car pulls up – a stranger yells, 'Get in, get in!' I jump into his car and we move off at speed. Safe, I think to myself, as I catch my breath, but as I turn and look out the back window I see that the horse is still chasing.

Even in the safety of that sanctuary, I see that the horse continues to pursue, refusing to give in. I look back and wonder what drives that beast on, what logic is at play, and the horse becomes something more than just a horse in my mind. It becomes some sort of metaphor for life.

We are all pursued. And sometimes we are saved. But one day the horse will catch up with all of us, when we are alone. And we are all alone at the end of the day. And it is then that we know who we really are. To accept this fact of life takes a great deal of strength. More than most people realise.

Overcoming

I always knew I was strong, I just didn't realise how strong I would need to be, especially on that day, 12 January 2018, when the horse finally caught me. Nothing could have prepared me for what happened next.

2

Making Memories

I HAD BEEN CANCER-FREE FOR more than three years and was used to the routine check-ups. Keeping an eye on things. Checking in every couple of months. My daughter Amelia was with me in the hospital. She had a separate appointment with her neurologist and that had all gone well. She was doing fine. That's all that mattered. I hadn't had time to think about my own appointment, until I was there, in the waiting room. Mam was with me too. Three generations, like ducks in a row – Amelia, me and Mam.

My cancer was back. I was there to find out about the treatment plan.

'Vicky Phelan, the doctor will see you now.'

I left Mam and Amelia in the waiting room. 'Won't be long,' I said, smiling towards Amelia. I took a seat in the consultant's room. I remember it was cold.

The doctor got straight to it. She told me it was not good news. She talked me through how the cancer had spread, with the aid of a diagram. I was trying to take it all in. But there was one question in my mind – could this be cured? I asked the doctor to tell me if I stood a chance. I could feel the weight of that question hanging in the air.

And then the answer: she told me that unfortunately, the cancer looked to be terminal. I asked her what kind of a timeframe I was looking at. I had to push her for a reply. I needed to know. With chemotherapy, I may have a year, at most. Without it, maybe six months. I was shocked. I tried to take it in. 'Surely there's something I can do?' I pleaded.

Radiotherapy was not an option because of the position of my tumours, which were close to all my vital organs. The only option available to me was to have more chemotherapy – palliative chemotherapy. I couldn't believe what I was hearing.

She was referring me to a medical oncologist who would discuss the chemotherapy plan with me. I asked about alternative treatments.

There were no options, it seemed.

What did this mean? I tried to make sense of it in my own mind. I was imagining the worst possible scenario: I had to go home, say goodbye to my children, and get my affairs in order.

I was furious. I had done everything they had asked me to do – I'd been to every gruelling treatment, and now, here I was three years later with terminal cancer.

I stared at her. I looked straight into her eyes, woman to woman. She looked down at the papers on her desk. 'Is that what you'd do? Give up? I have two children. I can't give up.'

With that I got up and left the room. The moment I heard the door close behind me, I put my hand out to steady myself against the wall. My legs were shaking. My head felt light.

There was a bathroom just to the left of the surgery, away from the waiting room. I stumbled in, and locked the door behind me. There was a sign on the wall that read, 'Call, Don't Fall'. And what did I do? I fell apart. I wept until there was nothing left in me. Everything was going through my head, and nothing.

Eventually, when I had no more tears to shed, I splashed my face with water and tried to gather myself. I couldn't let Amelia see me like this. I tried as hard as I could to seem normal. I put on my best face and went back to the reception area. But the moment Mam saw me, she knew. Mammies always know. She looked at me, over Amelia's head. 'Everything alright?' she asked.

I shook my head.

We made nervous chit-chat in the car on the way home, with Amelia in the back. As soon as we got in, Amelia went upstairs to her bedroom and I told Mam what the doctor had said.

That was over a year ago now, as I write these words.

I used to wonder how they could do it – people who had been told they didn't have long to live. How did they get up every morning? How did they keep going? I didn't understand it. Now I do. There's actually something liberating about it. When your days are numbered, you see the beauty of every day. It's almost like a second life.

And my second life began for me that day, when I stumbled out of the doctor's office. They say there's nothing more dangerous than someone with nothing to lose. I know who I am now, and what I need to do.

Everything that came next, after that day, everything you are about to discover, and all that came before it, was all for Amelia, and for Darragh. My children are what drives me, every day, and what makes me fight for any time I can have with them here on this earth.

I do not know how this book will end, or if I will make it to the end. But I need to tell this story, while I am here to tell it. While I have time on the clock. How this all came about. The secrets, the trials, the tribulations. And I swear I will tell you everything, as best I can. The unvarnished truth.

I am Vicky Phelan. And this is my story.

3

The Beginning

IT'S HARD TO BE SURE of your earliest memory. Things you actually remember, rather than are told.

I was born on 28 October 1974, in Airmount Hospital in Waterford city in the south of Ireland. My parents were living in County Kilkenny at the time.

I was Gaby and John Kelly's first child, and they were as excited as any young couple about to start a new family. They named me Vicky, Vicky Kelly. You've probably never heard of Vicky Kelly, but she was the makings of Vicky Phelan.

My mother was nineteen when she had me. And she went on to have four more children, three in quick succession.

While there was little by way of money when I was growing up, I never wanted for love and affection.

For the first five years of my life, we lived in a very rural part of Kilkenny, a place called Ballygorey, in a small cottage that my father fixed up before he and my mother got married. I remember the grass grew in the middle of the road and old wrought-iron gates marked the entrance to our home. The house was three miles from the village. It could be harsh at times. It was cold and damp in the winter time. But in the springtime, our garden filled with daffodils.

We were surrounded on all sides by fields, cut through by a dark ribbon of river, the River Suir.

My father knew every bend in that river. He was a fisherman. His family had fished the river for generations; the river was in his blood. He went to work each morning before dawn and wouldn't return until late at night. He practised the old traditional snap-net fishing where two boats row out onto the water trailing a net between them. They'd wait patiently, sometimes for hours, until the moment came, then row back in, closing the net, to reveal their day's catch. Then off to the fishmonger's in Waterford to sell the spoils.

Our lives revolved around the fishing season. And when the season was over, Dad had to find other work; he was able to turn his hand to most things. He had a lot of part-time jobs, mainly driving trucks and vans.

My parents were young, just making their way in the world, like most young couples do. My mother worked hard to make our house a home. She spent her days doing all the thankless tasks a mother tended to do: cooking and cleaning and minding the children. Their only car my father took to work, leaving my mother at the cottage alone all day with the children, miles from anywhere, with no mode of transport, except walking or cycling. Times were tough, but somehow they always managed to make ends meet.

It was here in Ballygorey that our family began. My earliest memory is from that time. It was the day I disappeared. My mother still talks about it, which must be why it has stayed with me. It is every parent's worst nightmare when a child goes missing.

It was 1978 and by that time my mother, at the age of twenty-two, had three very young children – me at the age of three, and the two babies, Robbie and Lee. That afternoon Mam was feeding the babies in the kitchen. They always ate first, then I would be called to sit at the table. Mam had a routine and it worked. Usually.

But this day was different because when it was my turn to be fed Mam called out to me from the next room as she always did. 'Vicky!'

But this time, no answer came.

'Vicky! Time for tea,' she tried again.

When there was still no answer, she hoisted the two little ones into her arms and went to look for me in the sitting room. My books and toys were scattered across the floor, as though I had just been there.

Mam went from room to room, calling my name. She looked under the beds and inside the wardrobes, checking all my usual hiding places. When there was no sign of me, she began to panic. She opened the back door and peered into the garden. Still no sign.

At the front of the house, she saw that the gate was ajar. It was always closed; they were always very careful to keep it that way.

With the weight of a baby in each arm, she ran as fast as she could towards my grandmother's house which was further up the road, hoping I might be there. She arrived at the house and raced up the garden path. 'Nanny Kelly?' she called. 'Mrs Kelly?' My grandmother was hard of hearing; you nearly always had to call her twice.

She was sitting on a bench in the back garden, potting flowers, when my mother appeared into view. 'Nanny Kelly, is Vicky here?'

'Hello, Gaby. What's wrong?'

'Is Vicky with you? She's not at the house. Did she come up here?'

'I haven't seen Vicky since yesterday.'

My mother's mind went to the worst possible place: the river. 'Will you take the boys for me? I need to find her.'

She placed the babies on my grandmother's lap, and ran out the gate. She passed our house on the right and continued down the road, towards the dreaded river.

From the moment they had moved to the cottage, the thought of the river being so close by had terrified my mother, especially with small children in the house. She couldn't swim and hated being near the water.

As she turned the final bend in the road that day, her mind was as dark as the river. Rounding the corner, she saw, coming up the lane towards her, the old man who lived in a thatched cottage on the far side of the water. And there beside him, wearing his old tattered cap, was me, followed in tow by my faithful dog, Bruce.

My mother was nearly too relieved to be angry. 'Jesus Christ, Vicky!'

'I found her sitting by the river, with the dog, missus,' the old man explained. 'I was bringing her back to you. I knew you'd be worried sick.'

'Thank you for finding her, Tom, and minding her for me.'

Standing beside my small frame, he must have looked like a quiet, gentle giant. The locals called him Tom 'the glasses'.

'You'd want to be careful with her going down to that river by herself – that current's mighty strong,' said Tom, wiping his glasses on the sleeve of his shirt.

'She managed to get out of the house again without me seeing her. I don't know how she does it.'

I could feel the tension as I was marched back home; I knew I had pushed the boundaries too far this time. But for my poor mother, this was just the start of it, the beginning of Vicky Kelly's adventures. There would be much more to come.

'We're in trouble now, Bruce,' I said.

Bruce wagged his tail, as if to say, *It'll be okay*. And I knew it would be. I couldn't help my natural curiosity, any more than I could help the colour of my eyes. And I felt my mother knew that too.

4

Mr Dineen

AT THE RIPE OLD AGE of three and three-quarters, I decided it was time for a major change in my life. I decided that I was ready for school.

Every morning I stood at the low window at the front of our house; I was just about tall enough to see out over the sill. I stood on my tippy toes and watched the older children from nearby houses heading off to school in the morning. I wanted to go where they were going – to Carrigeen National School. I begged my mother to let me go.

'You'll go next year, pet, when you're old enough.'

'Why can't I go now?' Always stubborn.

My mother had taught me to read. She taught us all to read very early on. I loved it and I couldn't see the point in waiting to join the great adventure of education.

'You're not old enough just yet. Be patient. Besides, there's plenty to do here in the meantime to keep you busy.'

I whined and whined, and eventually my mother gave in.

'Alright,' she said, 'why don't we go and speak to the headmaster. We'll see what he says.'

I couldn't believe it. This was my chance. The next day I woke up early; I had a lot to do that day. I immediately reminded Mam of her promise to go and see Mr Dineen.

'Alright, alright, we'll go this afternoon.'

My morning was spent picking out clothes to wear for this very important meeting. I needed to make a good impression. I chose my favourite jumper and a pair of blue tights. I laid my favourite reading books out on the bed. I would pack these and bring them with me. At ten o'clock, I was armed and ready to go.

Little did I know my mother had a plan. She was sure that I would be dissuaded by the headmaster, that he would tell me that I was too young to start school, and that would be the end of it. But I was ready for action.

I held my mother's hand as we walked through the school gates. I could see the boys and girls through the windows, sitting in rows, teachers standing at the blackboards. I could smell the musty scent of chalk in the corridor as my mother led me towards the headmaster's office. The walls were filled with children's paintings – colourful and bright. I couldn't wait to have my painting there too.

We reached the end of the hallway and knocked on the headmaster's big oak door.

'Come in!' said Mr Dineen.

We entered. A tall man sat behind a desk, peering out over bifocal glasses. My mother hoisted me up on to a large wooden seat.

'Well, hello, Mrs Kelly. Who do we have here?'

'This is Vicky. Vicky, say hello to Mr Dineen.'

'Hello,' I said, suddenly feeling very important in this unfamiliar atmosphere.

'I believe you are looking forward to starting school, Vicky?'

'Yes,' I said, looking down at my feet dangling over the edge of the wooden seat.

'How old are you?'

'I'm three,' I said, confidently. 'Three and three quarters. I'll be four in October.'

'Well, usually the boys and girls don't come to us until they are four years old. At least four.'

At this point, I decided there was nothing else for it. Much to my mother's surprise, I reached into the satchel and took out a book. I stood to my full height on the chair and began using the voice that my mother used when she was tucking me in at night.

'Once upon a time …'

My mother watched in disbelief.

'… in a land far, faaaar away there lived a little girl …'

I took a deep breath as I turned the page, which was a tricky manoeuvre considering I was trying to balance on the big wooden chair.

'Well, that's very impressive,' said Mr Dineen, looking greatly amused by the whole encounter.

I looked at him. He realised I was waiting for him to say something.

'Well, Mrs Kelly, contrary to what we might be led to believe, I think Vicky is ready for school.'

'She isn't four years old yet,' my mother reminded him. 'Don't you have to be four?'

'I know, but she is a very good reader. Who taught you to read so well, Vicky?'

'My mammy.'

'Well, she must be a very good teacher. Why don't we start you in baby infants and see how you get on?'

I started school the following Monday.

My mother told me this story recently. Just after my diagnosis. One of her earliest memories of me. I had never heard her mention it before, in all the years. She said it just came back to her. I think she told it to remind me of who I am, and who I have always been – determined, from a very young age.

It's funny, when you're nearing the end of your life, how you replay things from the beginning. Like me remembering that day with Bruce by the river, and being rescued by Tom 'the glasses' and my mother, even though I didn't know I was being rescued at the time. As a child, you expect to be rescued. It's as though life is a game.

But cancer is not a game. That's why you need rescuing in different ways. When my mother remembered that day in the headmaster's office, she was still coming to my rescue. By telling me that story, of the day I started school, she reminded me of my strength. She was still saving me.

5

School Days

MAYBE ONE RUN-IN WITH the River Suir was one too many for my mother, I don't know. But less than a year later my parents decided to leave Ballygorey. In the summer of 1979 we moved to a council house in Mooncoin, just a few miles away. It was a better place to be with a growing family, and my mother felt much less isolated. The village had a school, two shops, two pubs and a church. Everything you could need.

But it meant I would have to start school again, another first day for me.

The school in Mooncoin was much bigger than the one in Carrigeen that I had been in with Mr Dineen, which had just two classrooms and two teachers: one room for the junior classes and one room for the senior classes. Mooncoin Girls School on the other hand had lots of classrooms, each with their own teacher.

My parents worried the move would unsettle me, but I didn't seem to mind change. School for me was an escape. I got bored at home and needed the distraction of other children my own age. A girl called Maria sat next to me on my first day at the new school. We shared colouring pencils and soon became the best of friends, doing everything together. Little did I know that this was the start of a lifelong friendship.

The years passed and were full of the things that childhood brings – finding ways to use up all our excess energy, which usually involved getting into mischief. And a new brother and sister came along: Jonathan and Lyndsey. I finally had a sister. We were a band of five now, the Kellys, seven if you include Mam and Dad. Everyone loved coming to our house, including my best friends Maria and Susan, because it was full of fun and laughter.

We didn't have much by way of money, and what little we had needed to stretch a long way. But we never wanted for anything. What my parents didn't have in money they made up for in imagination. My mother baked, knitted and sewed. My father made toys for us to play with, cobbled together from old pieces of cloth and wood and metal.

Mam and Dad had a way of bringing magic to things. Every Halloween they turned the house into a world of weird and wonderful creatures. Dad had a smoke machine and puppets of ghouls and goblins and monsters that they hung from the ceiling. Every child in the village made the pilgrimage to see 'The Gruesome Grotto'.

At Christmas, the house was transformed into a winter wonderland, complete with Santa Clause, his reindeer and fairy lights. The excitement would continue to build until the big day, Christmas Day, our favourite day of the year.

Whoever woke up first on Christmas morning woke everyone else, and then we all clamoured down the stairs to see what Santa had left under the tree. My parents always locked the sitting-room door in order to build suspense. Dad would delay, on purpose, until our excitement was almost unbearable.

'C'mon, Dad!' we'd yell in unison. 'We want to see the presents!'

Finally, he'd turn the key slowly, like he was performing a ceremony, and we'd all fall into the room.

For the next couple of hours, the house was even noisier than usual, as we played with our new toys, running in and out of the house to show off some particularly valued item to our friends along the street. Then it was time for mass, and within half an hour, Mam and Dad managed to get us washed, dressed and presentable, and sitting quietly in the church, as if butter wouldn't melt in our mouths.

Those days of innocence passed very quickly indeed. And because I was the eldest, I got used to minding the others and taking responsibility, to help Mam and Dad get things done around the house.

By the age of twelve, as my primary-school days came to an end, I had a strong mind of my own and had a clear idea of where I wanted my life to go. I still had the tenacity of that three-year-old who stood in front of Mr Dineen.

There was a very good secondary school in Waterford, the Mercy, where Maria and some of my other friends were going and I decided that that's where I would go too.

'There's a perfectly good secondary school on our doorstep,' my father said. 'Why would you want to go further away?' He was referring to the Tech in Mooncoin, a vocational secondary school with a focus on practical subjects like woodwork and metalwork.

I argued with my parents for days. They insisted I was

going to the Tech, while I stubbornly extolled the merits of the Waterford school. After all, I was very academic.

'You're going to the Tech and that's the end of it,' my mother said in exasperation one day after we had been arguing all morning.

That evening, when my parents thought I was in bed, I crept out onto the landing in my pyjamas and overheard them talking in the kitchen. They were discussing whether they could afford to send me to the school in town. The uniform and the bus were the issue. They couldn't justify the expense of sending me to school in town when there was a school five minutes up the road from our house which didn't have a uniform. It would all add up, especially with four other kids coming up behind me. They were struggling with money and my mother was very worried about it.

At breakfast the next morning, Mam handed me a cup of tea. 'You know, if you really want to go to the school in Waterford, we might be able to find a way …'

'No thanks, Mam,' I said. 'I've changed my mind. Some of the girls from school are going to the Tech and, sure, I'll make new friends. It's a good school and it'll be good for me.'

The Tech was a mixed school, and I actually preferred that. I always found boys more straightforward, a consequence of growing up with three brothers. You knew where you stood with them.

I started at the Tech and was making friends and settling in. All was going well, until I found myself on Paula's radar. One day in the bathrooms while I was washing my hands, I looked in the mirror and saw her sitting on the toilet seat in the cubicle behind me, smoking out the window.

Paula was an older girl, two years ahead of me, with a tight ponytail and thick makeup. She was known for being a bully.

She caught my eye in the mirror and glared at me. 'What?' she said. 'Are you going to tell someone?'

'No,' I replied. 'I'm just washing my hands.'

From that day on, whenever she saw me in the bathrooms or in the corridor she pushed me against the wall or elbowed me as she was passing.

This went on for weeks. Until one day, when I walked into the bathroom and saw her perched on the toilet seat again, this time surrounded by her friends. She leapt up and gave me an almighty push. 'Look who it is!' she teased.

I could feel my anger building. 'Enough is enough!' I yelled, to the surprise of everyone, including myself. 'Paula, I'm tired of this. I think we should go down to the headmaster's office and talk this through.'

She froze on the spot. She wasn't good at talking. She liked pushing and shoving. I braced myself, expecting her to launch at me again. She gave me one last menacing look and returned to her throne.

I quietly breathed a sigh of relief. The mood had changed in the room. You could feel it. Her face was red. Her cronies could see she was shaken.

We never did go to the headmaster's office, but Paula never bothered me again from that day on.

I must have made a good impression, because when the bell rang that day to say that school was out, one of the older girls yelled over to me, 'You comin' down the pound?'

'Umm ...' I didn't know what that meant. 'Sure,' I said, chancing my arm.

She beckoned for me to follow her. The 'pound', it turned out, was the wall beside the village shop which served as both a bus stop and a hangout for the local kids. It became our regular haunt. We didn't do much there but sit on the wall and talk and pass the time the way teenagers do. Every day brought some new adventure: someone was 'shifting' someone new or some kind of row had broken out amongst the year. Always something to talk about.

They were still getting to know me in the group, but I could hold my own with the boys as well as the girls. I could take a slagging as well as the best of them. That seemed to give me credibility.

One day the boys had a hurley and sliotar and were playing puck-about at lunchtime. They were short someone to play, so I volunteered. I was running down the field when one of the lanky awkward lads accidentally fired the ball straight at me, striking me in the forehead and splitting my eye open. There was blood everywhere. One boy looked like he was going to pass out at the sight of it. Mr Buckley, one of the teachers, put me in his car and drove me to the hospital; I needed five stitches. We made it back before school was over, and I told Mr Buckley that I wanted to return to class, afraid that I would miss something. Before he could argue, I had marched back in for the remainder of the day.

My mother wasn't impressed when she saw me later that evening. 'What the hell happened to you, Vicky?' She scolded me as she tried to wash the dried blood that had matted through my hair. 'You're way too old for this kind of carry-on.'

I went into school the next day, holding my head high, displaying my war wound. It looked much worse than the day before. My eye was swollen, black and blue, but when everyone stopped to admire the vivid colours of the bruising, it sort of helped to take the sting away.

As the months wore on, even though I loved hanging out

'down the pound', the days were long sometimes and I knew deep down that I needed to focus on my studies if I was ever going to make something of my life.

I had Miss Keyes to thank for that. She was my French and English teacher. One afternoon, when she was handing back my French homework, marked with an 'A', she said to me, 'You know, Vicky, you'll go far in the world, if you just manage to stay focused.'

That had a big impact on me. She was the first person in my life to say something like that to me, to make me believe I could go somewhere, maybe even to college. She was my favourite teacher. That's not to say that she was easy on me; she could be very strict, and was constantly reminding me to apply myself. But she never forgot about me, always coming back to check in on my grades and to see if I was studying for the next exam.

She encouraged me to see the world too. Between my Junior Cert and Leaving Cert, she asked me if I would be interested in going abroad for a few weeks to work on my French.

'I'd love that!' I said.

She asked a friend of hers who lived in France to put up a notice advertising me as an au pair. And before long, someone answered: a family looking for a nanny to help take care of their two young boys. It was a perfect fit.

So off I went, at the age of sixteen. No mobile phone or email, just an address and handwritten letters. The family lived in Reims, a town in the heart of the Champagne region. I flew to Charles de Gaulle airport in Paris, where the mother of the family, Hélène, met me. She seemed friendly, and I tried as best I could to talk to her in French; I wanted to make a good impression. On our drive to Reims we engaged in small talk while I looked out the window, taking in the new surroundings.

'We're in the old town,' she told me as we turned down a cobbled side street and came to a halt. 'And here we are.' The house was like nothing I had ever seen before – a tall townhouse with a big archway, an ornate door and shutters on all the windows.

The housekeeper welcomed us inside. I placed my suitcase in the hall and looked up at the high ceilings and chandeliers and the old wooden staircase that curved upwards. Hélène showed me around the house. There were four floors and an interior courtyard filled with lush green plants. Everything was immaculately presented. She brought me through to the sitting room and introduced me to the children. The two little boys, Alexander and Benjamin, aged three and five, were playing on the floor. Their father wasn't there that day; he seemed to be at work a lot. She introduced the boys to me as their new English teacher, then brought me through to the kitchen to get to know me a little and outline my duties for the next few weeks. In the light of that room, I could take her in fully. She was glamorous and had an air that seemed kind and welcoming.

A great deal of my duties seemed to involve travel, which came as a very welcome surprise. Over the weeks I was there, I travelled with the family to Brittany to see the children's grandparents, and to Antibes, a coastal resort in the South of France they liked to go to for their holidays. We flew from place to place in the family's private plane. Their life seemed to revolve around swimming pools, exotic drinks, sunbathing and entertaining guests. And there I was in the middle of it all, a girl from a council house in Kilkenny! I really was a long, long way from home.

My job was mainly to speak English to Benjamin and Alexander and to get them ready for bed. When their parents were entertaining guests, as they often did, I went upstairs to read my book and kept an eye on the boys while they were sleeping, to make sure they didn't interrupt the dinner party. I enjoyed that quiet time on my own; I found the entertaining tiresome and shallow. Those in attendance were guests rather than friends, and I wondered what the point of it was. Though I liked to eavesdrop sometimes, from the stairwell, listening to their conversations to learn new phrases and vocabulary.

It was fascinating to witness another family from the inside, to observe how they operate. They were very different from my own family. They had everything they could want, but they didn't seem to have time for one another. The father was constantly on the phone, even when he was on holidays. The mother lounged around, generally looking unhappy, though it never seemed to draw the attention of her husband. Perhaps that's why she was unhappy.

I concluded that that kind of wealth came with a personality type. Their friends seemed to have a similar demeanour, though I couldn't imagine that they had much to stress about. They had cooks and cleaners and all kinds of people to do the things they didn't like doing. And they didn't need to worry about money.

I thought of my own parents, struggling to get by, trying to keep food on the table for five children at home.

When I arrived back in Ireland I bounded through the front door, taking in the familiar smells of cooking coming from the kitchen, and the football boots and school bags strewn about the hall, reminders of our chaotic life. My brothers clambered down the stairs and rounded on me with their usual witticisms and teasing. To their surprise, I hugged each of them as they passed, and did the same with my parents and Lyndsey who were in the kitchen. They seemed taken aback. My short time away had given me a new appreciation for what I had at home: my mad, wonderful family.

September came around and so another year of school. The Leaving Cert was the next major hurdle. It was going to be a big year for me and there were important decisions to make. I wanted to do well in the exams, but I didn't really know what I wanted to do after that. No one in my family had ever been to college. How did people know what course to apply for? How did you choose something that you would want to do for the rest of your life? It was overwhelming.

I decided to pay a visit to Miss Keyes; she would know what to do. She was sitting at the desk in her classroom marking papers. I knocked on the door.

'Vicky! Come in,' she said, leaning over the desk and pointing towards the chair in front of her. 'Please, sit down.'

'I was wondering if you could help me,' I said.

'In what way?'

'It's just ... I was thinking of applying to university.'

'I'm very glad to hear that.'

'It's just ... I don't know what to apply for.'

'Let's have a look, shall we?'

And with that she produced a brochure with all the courses that the University of Limerick had to offer. She sat with me for the next hour, as we leafed through the pages, talking about what interested me most and what I might like to do in the future.

'What about this one?' she asked, pointing at the European Studies course. 'You could do two languages with it.' It was an Arts degree that would give me the chance to work abroad again. It sounded perfect.

'Thanks, Miss Keyes,' I said, feeling relieved as I got up to go.

I had been feeling anxious, not knowing where I was headed in life. Now when people asked what I wanted to do after school, I would feel more confident about my answer.

This gave me something to aim for. I had a goal now and I pushed myself to get good grades. I taped colour-coded study timetables to the wall of my bedroom and created a flurry of Post-it notes and index cards, with nuggets of information to memorise.

When the big day finally came around I knew I was ready, but I was nervous all the same. As I walked towards the exam hall Miss Keyes smiled at me. 'Good luck!' she said as I passed her in the corridor.

The next few days felt like a blur. Exams followed by more exams, until it was all over and it was time to say goodbye to the Tech for good. Walking away, I felt grateful for the six years I had spent there. I was excited for what lay ahead, even though I didn't know what that looked like yet, or if I would be accepted into a university at all.

I spent the summer working, trying to make a bit of money. I went back to France to au pair for the same family. It was a good chance to practise my French, to give me a head start, if I was accepted onto the language course.

Towards the end of the summer the Leaving Cert results came out; I had the date marked in my diary for weeks. It was strange being away from home for such an important day. I was imagining everyone gathered at the school getting their results. I spent the day beside the pool in France, wondering when I would hear word from home.

Mam had promised me she would go in to see the headmaster to get my results. She went to my grandmother's house to phone me that evening. 'You got the best results in your class, Vicky! 460 points!' she said, full of excitement.

'What?!'

'Top of the class. The best results in the year,' she articulated slowly and carefully, making sure I could hear her.

I could hear her alright, but I couldn't believe it.

'The headmaster seemed surprised too!' Mam joked. We knew that people didn't expect much from kids from 'the street' – kids who didn't come from land or from parents with a professional background like a solicitor or doctor. My parents were working class.

'Ah, that'll show them! Thanks, Mam,' I said, suddenly feeling a weight leave my shoulders.

'Mam …' I paused for a moment. '… I only need 360 points for the course I applied for. You know what this means, don't you? I'll be going to UL in September.'

'I know, Vicky. Me and your dad are so proud of you.'

When the CAO results came out, I got my first choice – European Studies at the University of Limerick. I made it! I was going to college. The moment I was home from France, I went to see Miss Keyes to tell her the good news and thank her for her help.

'Well, Vicky, you did it!' she said, clasping her hands together. She seemed so happy for me.

I often wonder what my life would have been like if it hadn't been for Miss Keyes, pushing me the way she did, and Mam, constantly encouraging me to invest in my education. In a way, I think Mam wanted a life for me that she never had – a chance to make my own mark in the world, before marriage and family swept me off my feet.

6

Those Were The Days

THEY SAY YOUR SCHOOL DAYS are the happiest of your life, but for me it was my college days.

The whole concept of college was alien to me. I was the first person in my extended family ever to go to university. And I come from a big family – there are ninety-six first cousins on my father's side alone; he was one of sixteen children. So my going to third level was a big deal, for me, and for our entire family. I would be breaking the mould.

University wasn't discouraged, it just wasn't expected; it simply wasn't on the table. There were lots of things not on the table for people like me. We were working class and that's where we were supposed to stay, to man our station. At least that's how it felt.

And it was a strain, financially. College was going to be expensive. I prepared as best I could, spending the summer au pairing and waitressing to try to make enough money to get through the first term. The move to Limerick brought with it new complications, new costs, like where to live and how to pay the rent. By the time September finally came around I had saved just about enough to pay the registration fee and to buy the course books, and Mam and Dad had scraped together the money I needed for a deposit for accommodation. I don't know how they did it but somehow they found a way. They never let us down.

Dad drove me to Limerick the day before I was due to start college. The car was laden down with all my belongings and with enough food to keep me going for a month. 'Just in case you need it,' my mother said, squeezing another packet of pasta into the car. 'You never know.'

The first week at UL was called Orientation Week and was designed to settle the first-years in before the rest of the student population returned en masse. I was nervous. I had never felt so out of my comfort zone.

Dad reassured me that it would be okay. 'You'll be grand, Vicky. You'll find your feet,' he said. And with that, he left.

I sat in the middle of all my things from home, in this alien new place, a house-share in Limerick. Life was moving on quickly, I thought, and this was the start of a very different chapter.

The next morning I put on the clothes I had spent weeks picking out for my first day. It felt like the first day of school again. The campus was full of fresh-faced first-years trying to find their way around. You could sense the excitement in the air, the anticipation and the nervous energy of a fresh start, a new year, a new beginning for everyone.

I felt like, finally, I had arrived. Here were people like me, people who loved learning, who wanted to be here. Not like school, where you had to pretend you didn't, just to fit in.

The campus at UL was enormous. We had been given a map during Orientation Week. I took it out of my bag as I tried to find the lecture theatre for my very first Law lecture. The place was alive with the bustle of youth: that mixture of innocence and arrogance, when you feel invincible, like all the world's possibilities have been opened up to you.

As I walked through the door of the lecture hall, alongside all the other students, many of whom seemed to know each other, from school or somewhere else, for a moment I wished that Maria was there. We had been through everything together. I thought of the first day in Mooncoin national school when we shared our pencils. I felt as small as I did then.

I sat down, pulled out my notebook and pen, and got myself ready. I felt better being organised, having things set up. Ready to go. I was watching a couple who were sitting a few rows in front of me. They looked like a new couple, sitting side by side, whispering and laughing. I wondered what they were talking about, when I felt a tap on my shoulder.

'Sorry, is there anyone sitting here?'

I jumped; I had been miles away. I looked up. The boy standing beside me had jet-black hair and piercing blue eyes. I could feel the blood rush to my cheeks.

'Can I sit here?' he said, pointing to the chair beside me.

'Oh yeah, sure,' I said, awkwardly standing up, my notebook and pen falling to the floor. I stood out of his way and let him sit in beside me.

He was about to start a conversation with me, when the door opened and the lecturer walked in: a middle-aged man with a scholarly look about him, wearing a worn-out jacket and carrying a leather briefcase. His presence seemed to command attention. The moment he arrived, the talking in the room died down and all eyes fixed on him, including mine.

I am going to like it here, I thought to myself. And I did. I loved my lectures and worked hard at my studies. I joined clubs and societies and revelled in the nights out, late mornings in bed, new friends, boyfriends. People talking about ideas: old ideas tried and tested, and new ideas to be excited about. It seemed like anything was possible.

I was living in a shared house. I made good friends and we all lived in each other's pockets, popping over to one another's houses for cans of cider and spaghetti bolognaise. It's the best time – when you're finally an adult, able to make your own decisions, come and go as you please, but without the weight of real responsibility. I felt I had come alive, for the first time in my life. Like I finally had wings, and was flying my own course.

Maybe a little too much so. I know Mam worried about me, living away from home. She didn't have much of a sense of what I was up to, and when she saw me I was often recovering from a night on the town or coming or going from a party. 'I hope you study there as much as you seem to enjoy yourselves!' she would say when I was home for a visit.

And I knew she was right. By now I was in my second year of college, and it was time to get more serious about my studies. On 31 December 1993, I jotted down my New Year's resolutions in my old worn-out diary that I kept by my bedside.

Resolutions for 1994:
1. *Act more <u>responsibly</u> in my love life.*
2. *Cheer Up! Life is what I make it, myself.*
3. *Begin some serious exercise and lose weight for <u>myself</u>.*

4. *Be more sensible with my money.*
5. *Think of others before myself (especially Mam and Dad).*

There were things I knew I had to change. And 1994 was going to be the year to do it. Time for some growing up, I said to myself. I imagine most people have almost the same resolution list every year. We all want to be fitter, happier, kinder, loved and in love.

Some of my friends, including my best friend Maria, had boyfriends and were in relationships. I hadn't met anyone yet. I'd had lots of dalliances, but there was no one I had fallen for. Besides, I thought, a serious boyfriend would only be a distraction from college work.

I loved studying languages. They were like a secret door into another world, another culture. Learning a language was like decrypting a code. I felt I could be most expressive in French and Spanish. They brought out different sides of my personality.

By the end of my second year I was fluent in French, and my Spanish, which I had only started in college, was beginning to come on. One of the reasons I was so eager to go to UL was because of its work abroad programme, or Co-op programme, as it was called. UL was renowned for its Co-op programme across Europe.

It also had the largest Erasmus, or study abroad programme, of all the Irish universities. I was really excited about the prospect of working in France and studying in Spain to improve my competence in those languages, and to spend six months in each country deepening my understanding of the cultures and traditions and hopefully making some French and Spanish friends.

Having heard stories from students who had worked on holiday campsites such as KeyCamp and EuroCamp, I decided I didn't want to work in those places and I told the Co-Op Office that I would arrange my own work placement. So I contacted the family I had au paired for after my Leaving Cert year, knowing that if anyone could find me an interesting job, they could. They seemed to know everyone. They were delighted to hear I was returning. I made it clear that I wasn't coming back just to au pair, and they assured me that they would be able to find me something worthwhile.

I was giddy at the thought of being in France again. When I closed my eyes I could imagine myself back there: the light and the air seemed different, bright and soft. I could taste the cheese and wine; I could see the vineyards and the little cafés. I always yearned for France. In my mind it was a land where everyone rode bicycles in the countryside and the cities were sophisticated, with beautiful women and strong men, where people drank coffees, smoked cigarettes and had passionate love affairs. I knew it wasn't really like that, but I was ever the romantic. I couldn't wait to be back there.

With the little I had saved and with Mam and Dad's help I had just enough money to pay for the plane ticket. I felt guilty asking them for a loan, when I knew they had so little, but I promised to pay them back as soon as I was set up with a job in France.

Before I knew it, it was January and it was time to go. I carefully packed my suitcase with everything I thought I would need for six months away from home.

When the plane took off, it sent a rush of adrenaline through my body. I looked out the window and saw the green fields of Ireland getting smaller as we climbed high into the sky, away from land and up into the clouds. It was like magic, flying through the air. I always felt free when I was travelling.

Making my way through the airport in Paris, it felt great to be back in a place where French was the natural, everyday language. I was so used to hearing it in the classroom and reading it in books.

Having navigated my way through the Paris underground, I took the train to Reims, arriving a few hours later. I knew my way around, and got a taxi to the house in the old town. I was looking forward to seeing Alexander and Benjamin again. They must have grown a lot by now.

As before, the housekeeper greeted me at the door. She welcomed me in and helped me with my bag and brought me to the room on the third floor where I had been only a few years previously. It was a very familiar feeling to be back. A few hours later, the whole family arrived home; they had been visiting friends for the day. As they pulled up in the driveway, I was suddenly reminded of the hectic nature of life with them: kids screaming, parents scolding. My nostalgic memories very quickly faded away.

For the next few weeks I minded the children, fed them, put them to bed. Every day the parents told me they were very close to finding me another job. But as time wore on, I started to lose hope. I explained to them that I had come to France to practise my French in a more professional environment. Playing with children all day wasn't exactly stretching my vocabulary.

The weeks passed and I could see that no job was going to materialise. They were just happy to have an au pair again. So when the parents had gone to work one day I used the house phone to contact the university; I asked them if they had any placements available. I explained the situation and they said they'd look into finding me something. They would call back the following day. 'After twelve is perfect,' I said, knowing that the parents would be out at that time and I would be able to take the call.

The next afternoon a woman from the Co-Op Office phoned and told me they could set me up with a work placement they had in a hotel near Péronne, which was only a couple of hours away by train. There had been a cancellation, so there was a place for me – bed and board in return for forty hours' work a week.

I would work in the hotel as one of the interns, or *stagiaires* as we were called in France, for six months. There were two other students from UL there already, Mary Quinn and Lisa Murphy, along with other French and English students from hotel management courses. It sounded perfect.

An hour later someone from the hotel phoned to interview me. 'Hello, this is Monsieur Monceau.' He sounded very serious. 'Are you ready for the interview, now?'

'Emm … yes,' I said, tentatively. I was praying that neither of the children would come running in on top of me.

After a few minutes' conversation, Monsieur Monceau, who was actually the hotel manager, seemed satisfied that I would be well suited to the post and offered me the job.

'I'll take it,' I said, as I heard the kids arguing in the next room. I put down the phone and hurried in to restore the peace. This wasn't what I had signed up for, I thought, as they each argued their case. I was right to get out; I didn't want to be minding children for the rest of my life.

That night I told the parents that I would be leaving in two days' time as I had found alternative work somewhere else. They seemed surprised by the sudden announcement. It was a hard thing to tell them, but I didn't feel guilty. I knew that they had enough money to afford another au pair and that the children would be fine.

Two days later, I caught the train for Péronne. I felt a sudden sense of freedom, the adventure of setting off on my own again.

There are certain moments when life takes a turn, and often we don't even know that it's turning until we're looking back through the rear-view mirror. It's at those moments that the decisions we make can alter the course of our lives, for better or for worse. With retrospect you think, *What if I had turned left instead of right?* But at the time, all you can do is what feels right to you in that moment.

I looked out the window as the train trundled through villages, mountains and vineyards. Little did I know that the decision to go to Péronne would change my life forever.

7

Welcome To The Hotel Mercure

A S I EXITED THE TRAIN station, I heard a car horn. Parked just to the left was a little blue Citroën. In the front seat was a girl, a little older than me, with wild curly hair, glasses and a toothy grin. She was waving at me. 'Vicky?' she yelled.

'That's me!'

Her name was Marie. She was there to pick me up and bring me to the hotel. I climbed in.

'Thanks!' I said.

She clanked the car into gear. It stalled. 'Woops!' She started the engine again and fussed over the gears for a moment, and then we were off. 'Phew,' she said, smiling.

She was from the north of England, she told me, and had been working at the Hotel Mercure for a few months already. She was there with her friend Rachel. It was hard work, she said, but a lot of fun too. There was a good gang there and they all got on well together.

'Mary and Lisa are looking forward to having another Irish girl around,' she said. 'You'll be sharing a room with a French student called Katy so that should help improve your French. You'll have no trouble making friends! You'll fit right in.'

We pulled up outside the hotel, my new home for the next six months. *Bienvenue a l'Hôtel Mercure*, said the big blue sign outside the door. The building was six storeys high, built in a square shape with small windows and painted in bright vibrant colours. It had a retro seventies feel to it from the outside. It looked deserted. Inside, however, the décor was modern and the foyer was busy with the usual hum of a hotel lobby, with guests lounging in armchairs and staff serving teas and coffees. I tried to imagine myself in the same uniform serving the customers in a day or two.

Marie helped me to reception. 'See you later,' she said, putting down my bag and waving goodbye.

Muriel, the woman at reception, greeted me and showed me to my room. They had been expecting me. I followed her to the lift and up to the second floor. This was where all of the *stagiaires* were accommodated, she told me. 'Here we are,' she said, opening the door to room 210, my home for the next few months.

The room was large, with two king-size beds, a wardrobe and a dressing table. It looked to have everything I would need. For me, coming from a box room at home, it was heavenly. I had the room to myself, but would soon be sharing with Katy, from Lille, who was arriving in two weeks' time.

Muriel told me to unpack and to make myself at home, and to join them in reception whenever I was ready to have some food, meet the team and find out what tasks I would be responsible for. I unpacked my clothes and put them in the wardrobe and went to wash the journey off my face.

I always loved meeting new people, and this time was no different. But the anticipation of it I found nerve-wracking – knowing these would be my companions for the next six months and hoping I would like them and they would like me.

I went to the lobby and the manager who had interviewed me, Monsieur Monceau, greeted me and made the introductions. There were nine other students on work placement; they all gathered around to say hello. Marie was there and introduced me to her friend Rachel and to Nick, another hotel management student from Leeds University. Marie, Rachel and Nick would be in charge of supervising us. They were very chatty and immediately took me under their wing. I needn't have worried. The rest of the interns had been working at the hotel for a few months, so they seemed glad to have someone new in the mix.

I was assigned the job of manning the Bureau de Change desk as my French was better than that of most of the other English-speaking students. It was a much easier job than some of the more manual tasks in the hotel. I wouldn't be on my feet all day, though it did require a bit of mental arithmetic.

Lisa, Mary and I talked about who we knew back at UL, trying to find common ground. As it turned out, I knew one of Lisa's best friends, Sinéad, really well. We were in the same French class. We bonded over that and everything seemed very natural. We soon became firm friends.

When my new roommate arrived, I liked her from the moment I met her. 'I'm Katy,' she said, offering me her hand.

'Welcome to the Hotel Mercure!' I replied, wanting to pass on the goodwill of welcoming someone else to the hotel, taking her under my wing, until she settled in. Katy was younger than me; she was only sixteen. I couldn't believe that she was being sent on placement at such a young age. I showed her around and that night we stayed up talking for hours. She told me about her life, I told her about mine.

The following evening when we had finished up work for the day, I invited her to come for drinks with me and Lisa and Mary. We were going to the bar across the road from the hotel.

'Sounds great,' she said. 'Would it be okay if Christophe came along?' Christophe was a new hotel management student from Metz in the north-east of France who was working with Katy.

'Of course,' I said.

We gathered in the lobby. Katy was already there when we arrived, standing near the reception talking to a dark-haired boy.

'You must be Vicky,' he said as I approached. 'I'm Christophe.' He had dark brown eyes and a beautiful smile.

I shook his hand. 'Yes, I'm Vicky,' I said, feeling a bit shy all of a sudden.

I could feel there was a strong attraction. Throughout the night at the bar, we kept catching one another's eye across the table. As the night wore on we ended up sitting beside each other – a chance to talk privately. Talking with him was easy. We seemed to fall into a rhythm with one another. We were close in age and, though we came from different countries, we had a lot in common.

That night, as we walked back to the hotel Katy and the others went on ahead, leaving Christophe and me a few paces behind. As we were walking, side by side, he quietly slipped his hand into mine. I felt my stomach leap and my hands start to sweat.

We reached the door of my room and I could feel the tension building. Christophe turned towards me. Our eyes met and we kissed. Our first kiss. We both laughed a little afterwards, relieved to break the tension. He gave me a hug and a soft kiss on the cheek and went to his own room.

That night as I lay in bed, I replayed all of our conversations in my head. There was just something about Christophe that captivated me. He had a presence that drew me towards him. I couldn't stop thinking about him.

A few weeks later, a kiss turned into our first night together. In Christophe's room we talked and kissed through the night. He always had a way of making me feel special. I fell asleep in his arms. I woke to the sun beaming in through the crack in the curtains. I looked around. The bed was empty; Christophe was gone.

I decided to have a shower before making my way back to my own room. I sighed as the water moved through my hair and over my face; it felt reassuring and soothing. As I stepped out of the shower I heard the bedroom door open and close.

'It's me!'

'Christophe?'

'Breakfast!' he said as I emerged from the bathroom in my towel to find him sitting at the table with two coffees and two croissants. 'Good morning!' he said, smiling.

Over the weeks that followed this became a regular routine. We worked different shifts at the hotel so often we would only see each other in the evenings. His shift was early in the morning, so he got up at 6 a.m. A few hours later he would sneak away from work for a few minutes to gather some things from the hotel breakfast and bring them up to me on a tray while I was sleeping. I'd wake to find it by my bedside. And on the tray tucked away between the orange juice and a slice of toast or croissant would be a little note. He left one every day. A note to say hello or to tell me I was beautiful. He was a real romantic.

No one had ever shown love to me like that before. He was gentle, always checking to see if I was okay, or what he could do to make me feel happy. I felt protected, loved in a special way, for the first time in my life. And I loved being around him.

As spring became summer we grew closer and closer. But all the while, the thought that the summer would end, and we would have to go our separate ways, was hanging over us. It was the unspoken thing. Both of us afraid to get too close, in case we got hurt.

One evening in the bar, Christophe, out of nowhere, turned to me and said, 'How about I come and see you in Ireland … maybe meet your family and your friends.'

'Yes!' I said immediately. I loved the idea of it. Part of me needed the reassurance that this wasn't just a fling, that he was truly feeling what I was feeling. This was his way of telling me. It was instantly liberating. We could be as close as we liked. This was a relationship.

We spent that night in the bar talking about his trip to Ireland and all the places and people I would take him to see. We laughed as we played all of our favourite songs on the jukebox with Katy and Mary and Lisa. We were inseparable, the five of us – doing everything together.

In that moment, I looked around me and felt utter happiness. I wanted to press pause, and live in that summer for a lifetime.

8

Le Moment Tout A Changé

EVERYTHING IN LIFE HAS ITS season, and our season in France was slowly coming to an end. Katy was leaving for Lille the next day and soon we would all be departing. We decided to celebrate, to have one last night together, to see her off in style.

Someone from the hotel suggested a club in Albert, which was a bigger town some ten miles away. They said it was the best place to be on a Saturday night. It was a little further afield than we had been before; we usually went to the bar in Péronne. But this was a special occasion – the last hurrah of the summer. So we got dressed up and off we went. There were ten of us, so we travelled in two cars, driven by Christophe and Jean-Pierre, another French intern.

We danced through the night, lit by the fluorescent red and green scattered lights reflecting from the disco balls hanging from the ceiling as the DJ pumped out the tunes. Katy was in the middle of the circle as we danced around her and cheered her on. We'd miss her – she was always the life of the party.

We danced into the small hours of the morning. Then when it started to look like things were wrapping up, Christophe yelled, 'Let's head home!' The music of the club was drowning out his voice. I took his hand and he pulled me through the crowds as we made our way past the DJs and across the dancefloor to the exit.

Katy and Lisa were outside, smoking and talking with Chris Thomain, another hotel management student from Brittany, who was also trying to round everyone up to go home. It was 4 a.m. and some of us had to be in work in two hours.

'Ready to go?' they asked.

'*Oui, oui,*' I said, as we all moved towards the car, chatting loudly, and recounting stories from the night. We were joined by the other group from the hotel. Between us all, there was a lot of laughter and conversation.

'We have space in our car if one of you wants to join us,' said Mary as the other car filled up.

'I can go with you,' said Katy. But after a moment's discussion she decided to come with us instead, to finish off our last night together.

We piled into the car, Christophe at the wheel, me beside him in the passenger seat. He leaned over and kissed me. 'Let's go!' he said.

In that moment I felt a strong connection to him, and to my new life in France, a world away from Mooncoin, where I had grown up. I had never felt so happy. I felt like this was the life I was meant to live. I felt so alive.

'Turn it up!' they called from the back. Someone was smoking a cigarette out the window. I cranked up the radio. The DJ was playing French pop music and we all sang along loudly, yelling the chorus in unison. Those songs were the anthems to our summer. We knew them off by heart.

We were just three miles from home when in the distance we saw two bright lights. They looked to be heading straight for us. They were getting closer and closer and gathering speed. 'Christophe!' I screamed as something came hurtling towards us.

There was the sound of the screeching of brakes and then a crash. I felt a piercing pain and the feeling of a heavy weight against my body. A strong smell filled the air; the acrid smell of petrol.

Then everything went dark.

In my grandmother's house in Mooncoin, the Sunday fry had just been cleared away from the table. 'We'll leave in ten minutes,' Nanny Fitzgerald called down the stairs to my aunts Tina and Ann who were finishing a cup of tea. She didn't like to be late for mass.

The phone rang.

'I'll get it!' said Ann. 'Hello.'

The voice on the other end spoke in broken English, with a strong French accent. Ann found it difficult to understand, but one thing was for sure, he said the words 'Vicky Kelly'.

My aunt looked anxiously towards Tina and motioned for her to fetch a pen and paper. She scribbled down the details as best she could. Her hand was shaking. 'An accident? What did the doctors say?'

My grandmother walked into the room. She and Tina listened intently to the conversation.

'Is Vicky okay?' She listened closely to the reply. 'Thank you,' she said, slowly, as the caller's English was limited. 'We will get there as fast as we can.'

Ann put down the phone. 'It's Vicky,' she said. 'There's been a terrible accident. We need to tell Gaby and John.' She got into her car and raced towards my parents' house, less than half a mile away. She rang the bell and my mother came to the door. Immediately she knew there was something wrong.

'Ann, what is it? Is it Mammy?'

'No, Gaby. It's Vicky …'

'Oh Jesus. John!' She called for my father, who was at the back of the house. 'John!'

'Ann, what's happened?' she said.

'Let's go inside and sit down,' said Ann, taking my mother's arm and guiding her towards the living room.

My father entered the room looking worried. 'Something's happened to Vicky,' my mother told him in a hurried, anxious tone.

'You had better sit down,' Ann said. 'A man called a few minutes ago. Vicky's been in a serious car accident in France. She survived.' She paused, letting that information sink in.

'Some of the others in the car didn't survive. But she did. She's in hospital in a place called Amiens and they are operating on her today.'

My parents looked stunned. The colour drained from my mother's face. My father put his arm around her.

'We need to get you to France,' Ann said. 'I'm going to go back to the house and organise passports and flights. Pack enough to keep you going. You might be there for a good while.'

She hugged my mother. 'It's going to be okay, Gaby. She's going to be okay. But she needs you now so we are going to get you over there as soon as we can, okay?'

My father walked to the door with Ann. 'How is she, Ann?' he asked, quietly. 'Did they say?'

'It doesn't sound good. We need to get you there. You pack some things and I'll be back shortly.' She squeezed my father's hand and left.

A few hours later Ann had organised for two emergency passports to be issued and for my parents to fly to France that evening.

My Uncle Frankie and Aunt Kathleen decided that they would go with my parents. Frankie drove. The atmosphere was tense as the car creaked and clanked. The engine had been acting up. Every few miles, it sounded as if it was going to cut out. My mother looked nervously at my father. They needed to make it to the passport office in time to collect the passports and get to the airport. My parents were worried. They had never travelled abroad before and were leaving behind four children including my sister Lyndsey, who was only nine years old. They were full of the apprehension of flying, never having been in a plane, and more so what they would find when they arrived, not knowing if I would survive the operation.

After what felt like a long drive to Dublin and a stop-off at the passport office, they made it to the airport just in time. Slamming the car door shut, my uncle muttered that he'd like to leave the heap of junk in the parking lot for good. It had been touch and go whether they'd make it or not.

They rushed through the airport and boarded the flight, with only minutes to spare.

9

The Aftermath

'WHERE IS SHE?' MY MOTHER asked, as she rushed through the hospital doors. I was in the intensive care unit.

Katy's mother, Sarah, was at the hospital and saw my parents arriving in distress. She hurried over to help translate as she could see my parents were struggling to understand. The doctors were trying to explain that I was in an induced coma and they would not be able to see me.

'I need to see Vicky,' Mam said sternly, determined that strangers were not going to stand in her way. 'Where is she?'

Sarah spoke with the doctors, and after a few minutes' discussion they agreed to take my parents to see me. They gestured for Mam and Dad to follow them, and led them down a long corridor. The doctors continued to speak in French, even though my parents could not understand. They were glad to have Sarah there with them. She was British, but spoke fluent

French. They felt a long way from home. How life can change so quickly.

They entered a room filled with monitors, with black and white images on each of them.

One of the doctors pointed at a screen. 'Vicky,' he said.

My parents looked confused. They had been expecting to arrive at my bedside and thought there must be some misunderstanding.

'Vicky,' the doctor emphasised again, pointing at the monitor. Mam and Dad examined the image on the screen, trying to make it out. All they could see was my mummified body, covered from head to toe in bandages, with two black eyes and plasters all over my face: cut, bloody and raw.

'That can't be her. John, that can't be Vicky,' said my mother, watching the monitor in disbelief.

No part of me was recognisable. I was in a coma. I had severe internal bleeding so the doctors had induced the coma, to see if they could stabilise me. They told my parents there was no way of knowing if I would come out of the coma alive.

Every day my parents came to look at the monitor, searching for signs of life. Agonising over the image for the slightest movement. None came. They waited and waited. And then, after nearly a week, I woke up.

People think coming out of a coma is like waking from a deep sleep. It's not. It's very frightening. It's like emerging from deep waters. It is disorientating and confusing. And the mind plays tricks on you, as it's full of medication.

As I opened my eyes, I began to hallucinate. I was seeing images on the ceiling of a man in a wheelchair, coming towards me. He was naked and his face was gnarled. He was getting faster and faster as he came closer. I thought he was going to rape me. I screamed. The doctors ran over. I felt hands pressing down on my body and someone injecting me with something. Suddenly I felt calmer.

I opened my eyes again and saw my mother and father beside me in the hospital room.

'Vicky …' My mother took my hand. 'We're here Vicky,' she said. 'Everything is okay.'

I could tell she had been crying. I was confused. I couldn't work out where I was, or why my parents were there. I tried to sit up and felt a searing pain down my back. I suddenly realised that I couldn't move my arms or legs. I looked down at my body. It was covered in bandages. 'Where am I?'

'You're in France,' said my father, 'in hospital.'

'Try and rest, pet. We'll tell you everything later.' My mother stroked my hand.

I could feel myself falling in and out of sleep. A heavy tiredness came over me.

I was very weak, but that was to be expected, the doctors said. As the days passed I became a little stronger. The consultants who checked in regularly seemed happy with my progress, which was a great relief to my parents. They could see signs of my personality coming back as I gained more energy.

The machine beside me beeped to signal it was coming to the end of its cycle. A nurse arrived and changed the fluids, resetting the machine. It was all becoming a regular routine.

Dad was sitting beside my bed, keeping vigil, as he did every day. I waited for the nurse to leave, for it to be just the two of us. 'Dad, what happened?' I asked, finally able to think straight. I couldn't piece it all together – how I had ended up in a hospital bed.

Dad looked as though he had been expecting this moment. 'There was an accident,' he said. 'You were going home with your friends from a nightclub – you and Christophe and Lisa and Katy and Chris Thomain.'

I was trying hard to remember. I could see Dad was trying to tell me something.

'Try and rest, pet,' said Mam, coming back into the room, feeling my forehead.

'Where is Christophe?' I asked.

They looked at one another for a moment, and I knew.

'Dad, what's happened to Christophe?'

Dad cleared his throat and squeezed my hand. 'I'm so sorry, Vicky ...'

'What are you saying?' I could feel the tears forming in my eyes.

'He was ...' He couldn't bring himself to say it.

I looked at him, pleading. 'Tell me.'

'Christophe was killed in the crash, Vicky.'

I could hear the words but they didn't feel real.

Dad cleared his throat again, in the way he does when he's nervous about something. 'Lisa,' he said, looking for a sign of recognition in my eyes, '... she didn't make it either.'

'What about Katy?' I asked.

'She's in intensive care. It looks like she might be paralysed, though it's too early to tell. Katy's mother is praying for a miracle.'

I felt like I was going to get sick. The blood drained from my face and I felt numb. I tried to move and remembered that I couldn't. Tears rolled down my cheeks. Even crying hurt, as my bruised and broken ribs made it impossible to catch my breath.

My mother came to my side and held my hand. It was all

she could do to comfort me. 'We were so worried about you,' she said. 'But you're going to be alright, Vicky. It's going to be alright.'

It didn't feel alright.

The days that passed were almost too much to bear. I didn't know how I would keep going. And yet I was trapped, in the casket of my bandages. Unable to move.

I've never felt so close to death in my whole life. I spoke to death, dared it to come, and began wishing for it. I could not cope with the burden of having survived when Christophe and Lisa had not.

I tried to piece things together in my memory. I remembered being in the car with the music playing. We were singing. Then we saw headlights coming towards us, getting closer and closer until they were blinding, followed by the crash, the darkness and the strong smell in the air. Then a loud noise which sounded like it was all around me.

'That was the helicopters,' Dad told me.

'Helicopters?'

My parents told me what they had learned from the police. It was after 4 a.m. A man was driving towards us on the wrong side of the road. Christophe turned the wheel to veer sharply to avoid the collision, but the man in the car veered too and went straight into us. Then the silence and the smell of burning flesh and petrol.

An off-duty fireman on his way home from work had veered a short time earlier to avoid the same car. From his rear-view mirror, he saw the flames from the crash and hurried back to the scene. He pulled over and ran towards the two cars. In one he saw a man slumped over the steering wheel; in the other he saw five young people. Time was critical. He had to choose which car to go to, who to save. He ran towards our car. I cannot imagine what he must have witnessed.

Christophe was dead in the driver's seat. There was no headrest in the car, so he was killed instantly by the impact. The rest of us were unconscious but still breathing. The fireman signalled for help on his radio.

He had seen these kinds of accidents before. He knew it was only a matter of time before the car caught fire. One by one he tried to pull us from the wreckage. He lifted me out, but my leg was twisted and stuck under the metal. He pulled and pulled, determined to free me before a fire broke out.

Two rescue helicopters, a fire truck and an ambulance arrived on the scene and rushed us all to hospital.

Lisa was severely brain-damaged and was in a coma for a week before her parents had to make the decision to turn off her life-support machine. She died on 17 July 1994. She was twenty-one.

Katy survived but was paralysed from the neck down. She was only sixteen at the time of the accident.

Chris Thomain, the other French student who was in the car, also survived. His legs were broken in several places and he had a bad cut on his head.

My injuries seemed to be in every part of my body. I broke my left ankle in three places, my left thigh, six ribs, my collar bone, my nose, my left cheekbone and I shattered my pelvis. I also had internal bleeding so I was left with a large scar on my stomach following a laparotomy where they had to cut me open to stem the bleeding. The laparotomy revealed that I had suffered damage to my kidneys. I also had to have skin graft surgery on my left ankle, as the off-duty fireman had to wrangle me out of the burning vehicle, leaving part of my ankle behind.

I was unconscious for a week. No one thought that I would survive. Deep in my heart I knew Christophe was with me that week, watching over me and helping me get through it.

My wounds would heal, but the hardest part was knowing I would never see Christophe or Lisa again. I couldn't stop crying. I was exhausted from all the emotion.

I had a recurring nightmare. Christophe was there, but then all of a sudden he was gone. In my dream he was cheating on me. I could see him, but I couldn't connect with him. It felt like he was a different person. In the dream I kept reaching for him, but he was cold and aloof.

I chased after him, until eventually I stopped chasing and became angry with him. Then I confronted him. I couldn't believe he could throw away all that we had. I woke in a sweat, crying again. The dream was vivid. He had been there with me, and not there at the same time.

It was strange to have that dream etched in my mind. Even though it was all in my head, it felt like a memory, the feelings were real and yet they felt so foreign to me. I had never been angry at Christophe. He died before we ever had a cross word. He was perfect. And always will be.

I was due to be transferred to a hospital in Ireland in two weeks' time, having spent three weeks in Amiens hospital in France. The staff were trying to stabilise me so that I would be able for the journey home. I was counting down the days. I needed to get away from France to try to come to terms with what had happened. I wanted to be surrounded by my family and friends, by people who knew me and loved me.

I looked at my diary. It was Saturday, 30 July – I was trying to work out why the date felt important, and then I remembered. In my purse were two Pink Floyd tickets for that date at the Château de Chantilly, Chantilly Castle. Christophe and I had planned to go to the concert together. Just three weeks previously we had talked excitedly about the kind of day we would have – about travelling to Chantilly by train, the thrill of seeing the band live on stage, where we would stay, what we would do. It was going to be our first trip away together.

I should have been in Chantilly with Christophe at the concert. Instead I was lying in a hospital bed, nearly paralysed, unable to do anything except blink and move my arms. And Christophe was dead. I closed my eyes and thought of the tickets in my purse. Two tickets. Two empty chairs at the concert.

For the first time in my life, I knew what love felt like. And how much it could hurt – really hurt. I missed Christophe every day. I kept thinking he would come through the door. I imagined his smile, I could almost hear his voice. It hurt the most when I reached for him and couldn't find him.

I hadn't completely lost my faith in God, but I couldn't make peace with it either. Why us? I felt God was the reason I was alive; He had saved me. But was it worth it? I knew I shouldn't think that way, but I couldn't help it. I couldn't see the point anymore, of life, when people could be taken away so easily, without reason. Why did He take them? They didn't deserve it.

All these things were going through my mind as I was waiting to go down for another operation in the 'bloc', as they called it. Another skin graft on my ankle.

As I waited in that vacuum of time, before the nurse wheels you into the operating theatre and you are put to sleep, I prayed for two things at once. I asked Christophe and Lisa that if I made it back I would be free from the awful pain. And then I prayed to God that He would just take me, on the operating table. On condition that I would be with Christophe. Life and death basically meant the same to me. I used to be afraid of death but now, I wished for it. It would bring me closer to Christophe.

A few hours later, I woke up back in the ward. I was in agony. I had offered it up to God – a second chance to take me, and He hadn't. I took it as a sign, a sign that I needed to make the most of the life I had been given. But it was going to take a long time to learn how to live again. Death still roamed my head most of the time. I was always thinking about it.

I organised for a bouquet of flowers to be sent to Christophe's parents as Sunday marked a month since the accident. I missed him every day. I smiled as I remembered how he used to say, *'Fait ton grimace pour moi, s'il tu plait, Vicky.'* ('Make that face for me, please, Vicky.') Except that I couldn't make that face anymore, the one that he loved, where I scrunched up my nose and pursed my lips, and then he would give me a kiss. I couldn't do it anymore, with my broken nose and cheekbone.

So that face will always be for you, Christophe.

10

The Bend For Home

J ULY WAS HOT AND HUMID. The hospital windows
were open and the fans were working hard to keep cool air
moving through the wards.

Mam and Dad were finding it hard to cope with the heat.
Every day they walked to the cathedral in the middle of Amiens
to seek refuge from the high temperatures. They picked a pew and
sat there for an hour or so, enjoying the cool air of the church.

One day, when they were approaching the steps of the
cathedral, my mother suddenly collapsed on the pavement. My
father called for help, in his best broken French, '*Au secours!
Ma femme, ma femme!*' ('Help! My wife, my wife!')

He pointed frantically to my mother, lying on the pavement,
waving down passers-by for help. A man stopped and ran to
the nearest café to phone an ambulance. My father placed my
mother's head in his lap and tried to talk to her. She was coming
to but seemed a little confused. Then a van pulled up beside
them, and six men dressed in black bundled out.

For all the world, my father thought they were being kidnapped, and wondered what he might have said in French to illicit such a reaction. The men in black turned out to be paramedics. They were the SAMU, French emergency medical service personnel.

Back at the hospital a nurse rushed into my room to see me. My aunt and uncle, Kathleen and Frankie, were sitting beside my bed, keeping me company. The nurse was trying to tell me that my mother had been admitted to the hospital, and was in a bed two floors below me. She was speaking in French.

'Hospital?' I asked, not at all sure that I was hearing her correctly. 'What happened?'

'Dehydration,' she said.

And with that I burst out laughing. My mother was known for never drinking water. 'I'll be grand,' she would say when we tried to encourage her to do so. She only drank tea, and it was far too hot for tea, and she hated the UHT condensed milk you get in France. My ribs hurt with laughter, but I couldn't stop.

'What is it?' my aunt asked, looking very confused.

'It's Mam. She's in hospital,' I said, trying to catch my breath.

'What? Why is that funny?'

I finally settled down and told my aunt what had happened. My mother quickly recovered and was back on her feet the next day. But it was a lesson she didn't forget. For the remainder of our time in France, she was never to be seen without a bottle of Orangina.

A few days later, the doctors announced it was time for me to go back to Ireland; I was strong enough to be transported.

I could see Mam and Dad were relieved. They were ready

to go home. Mam packed my things; the Hotel Mercure had transferred my belongings to the hospital. Around my bed were soft toys and cards posted from Ireland by family and friends. Mam took them down and placed them one by one into the suitcase.

I could see that Mam was keen to get home. She was missing the three boys – Robbie, Lee and Jonnie – and my little sister Lyndsey. It had been five weeks, the longest she had ever been away from them. Mam and Dad were relying on letters and the occasional phone booth telephone call to check in on Lyndsey and the boys, who were being minded by my aunts.

'You will be leaving in the morning,' the doctors told me.

I tried to imagine what it would be like to be back in Ireland. I wanted to be home, in familiar surroundings, but it would be a while before I could savour the comfort of my own bed. The plan was to transfer me to a hospital in Waterford, until I regained my mobility.

The next morning I woke up feeling excited – for the first time in a long time. Instead of my daily routine, today was different. I was going home. I couldn't wait to breathe in the cold, fresh Irish air and to see my brothers and sister and my friends.

Mam and Dad arrived early that morning, bags packed and ready to go. As I watched them walking towards the bed, seeing them in such a different environment made me view them in a new light. They were a team, taking on whatever life threw at them. This was worlds away from the life they were used to, but they were doing it, for me. I felt very lucky to have them by my side.

'Morning, Vicky,' Mam said, and she bent down to give me a kiss on the forehead.

'Morning.'

'Ready to go home?' asked Dad.

'Am I what! You'll miss the French wine though!' I joked.

He'd developed a taste for it over the past month. They had been staying at the family accommodation attached to the hospital where they were given breakfast and dinner. And, of course, being France, dinner came with a pitcher of red wine. My father never drank anything except Guinness at home. By the end of the five weeks, he had become a fan of the *vin rouge*.

One of the nurses dropped by to check my blood pressure. 'Have they given you a release time?' she asked.

'Not yet,' I said. Everything always seemed to take longer than it should.

At that moment one of the head nurses came in. 'I have bad news,' she told me.

We all looked at her.

'What is it?' said Dad, sounding concerned.

'They seem to have had a problem organising the plane for today. It won't be possible to travel.'

I translated for my parents. I could see the disappointment in their faces. I felt somewhat responsible, though there was nothing I could do. The nurse explained that they needed to organise for a hospital bed to be fixed into the plane, which required some of the seats to be taken out. It was something that was done regularly, but it needed to be organised on the ground at the airport, and somehow, some part of the logistics had gone wrong.

'We really need to get home to our children,' said Mam.

The nurse didn't seem to understand. I repeated in French what Mam had said.

'Hopefully we will have something tomorrow,' she said, and left the room.

We all looked at each other. Life in France had taken on its own routine, and we had all got used to it, out of necessity. But we were excited about going home, so having to spend even one more day away left us deflated.

We chatted it through and decided that Dad, Kathleen and Frankie should go ahead and catch the flight we were supposed to be on and get everything set up at home and that Mam would stay with me and we would travel home together the following day.

The next morning I woke up a little less confident about what the day would bring. It felt like déjà vu. Mam arrived, bag packed and ready to go once more. We waited for an update from the medical team, who confirmed that we would be on our way in an hour's time. We were both relieved.

They began the process of discharging me, and when the ambulance was ready they lifted me carefully from one bed to another and wheeled me down the corridor. The wards were busy with people visiting, doctors attending to patients, patients trying to make the most of things. Just like us, I thought. So many different lives, gathered together, for different reasons. All trying their best. We are the lucky ones, the ones who can leave the hospital, I thought, thinking of Lisa who had died there only a few weeks before. Her journey out of there was in a coffin.

We were transported via ambulance to Paris. I was laid out in the back on a stretcher, Mam sitting beside me. I could feel every bump in the road, every pothole. I grimaced with the pain. 'Not far now,' Mam said, encouraging me as we went, though I could see the strain on her face.

When we arrived at Charles de Gaulle airport the paramedics seemed agitated. They were on the phone arguing about something. I could only hear bits of the conversation, but from what I could make out, it had to do with the aircraft insurance.

After a few minutes, the ambulance came to a stop and a paramedic appeared at the back door. 'There's been another delay,' he explained, looking fed up with the situation.

'What does that mean?' Mam asked me, concerned.

'You will have to stay in Paris this evening and they will try the transfer again tomorrow,' the paramedic said, with a sympathetic look. I could tell it was not his fault. We had no choice but to go along with it. Mam was nervous being in a foreign city for another night without Dad, but she had me.

They brought us to a hospital on the outskirts of Paris. It was very different from where we had been. Outside, the city streets were loud with traffic and wailing sirens. The noise was constant.

It was late, close to midnight by the time we were admitted. I was placed in an empty ward for the night. A nurse arrived with instructions for my mother to go to the family accommodation down the street. On her own. She looked petrified at the thought.

'Absolutely not, she's staying here with me,' I piped up from the bed.

'That's not possible,' said the nurse, sounding indignant at this interruption of procedure. 'This is for patients only.'

I looked around at the empty beds in the ward. 'Why can't she sleep here?' I pointed to the bed next to mine. I knew my mother wouldn't be comfortable walking the Paris streets at midnight.

I continued to argue with the nurse, who then brought a doctor in for back-up. I stood my ground and advised them to get in touch with the insurance company if they had an issue, since they were the ones at fault. She was staying in the ward, and that was that.

Eventually they gave in. Mam changed into her nightdress and got into the bed beside me. She looked exhausted from the day. We said goodnight, and turned out the light. Neither of us slept much, drifting in and out of disturbed sleep. The air was humid, sticky and hot. The noise of the sirens, and of hospital trolleys with squeaky wheels clanking along the corridor, made deep sleep impossible.

I woke to the sound of my mother crying. 'Mam? Are you okay?' I said, unable to turn in the bed towards her.

'I'm fine, pet,' she sniffled. But I knew she wasn't.

A siren sounded outside the window. The flashing lights lit up the ceiling, blue and red, just for a moment, and then they were gone. I could hear Mam crying again. 'It's going to be okay, Mam. I promise. It'll all be okay.'

I could feel the tears rolling down my cheeks. I hated that she was so upset. I was trying to turn in the bed but my body was in agony from the journey. I couldn't move. I could only speak to her softly in the darkness of the night, and hope that we would both get some sleep soon.

With tired heads we woke to the news that we would finally be going home. They brought us by ambulance to the airport tarmac. It took several men to lift me up the stairs of the aircraft, carefully manoeuvring the stretcher. People watched on inquisitively as they queued to board.

Once inside, they laid me down in the carefully prepared bed, strapped a seatbelt over me and asked if I was comfortable. It was an unusual feeling to be lying down in the aeroplane cabin facing the ceiling. As the passengers filed in, I looked up at them as they passed by. They averted their eyes, pretending not to look at me.

Mam sat beside me and held my hand. I was so impressed by her, how bravely she took it all in her stride.

There was something about being back in Ireland that felt reassuring. The colloquial greetings and jovial banter from the paramedic staff as they lifted me back out of the plane and into the ambulance made me feel at home. I felt more comfortable in Ireland, and so did Mam. It was hard for her to interpret each situation in France, without being able to speak the language. At least in Ireland she could gauge what was happening.

They transported me to Waterford Regional Hospital. It was a step closer to home, but still a long way from normal life resuming. That evening, I lay in my hospital bed, taking in my new surroundings, on my own for the first time in a long time. I usually tried to put a brave face on when Mam and Dad were around, as it was hard enough for them to cope. When I was alone, I could let my mind escape.

I watched a starling appear at the window sill, sit for a moment, and then fly away, becoming engulfed by the colours of dusk in the summer sky. I was deep in thought. Now that I was closer to home, I felt like I could let go again. I could feel the tears rolling down my cheeks. It was going to be very hard to try to live once more. I felt like I was starting from scratch. The thought of it was exasperating. I was already exhausted.

I made the decision there and then: no matter how hard it would be, I needed to live fully, for Christophe and Lisa, who never got a chance. I'll do it for them, I thought. I looked up at the ceiling and said thank you to Nanny Kelly, because I didn't think I could have made it on my own. She had passed away three years before, and I knew she had been watching over me.

The first step in continuing to live was learning to walk again. I was exhausted from all the emotions, all the crying. But I was also physically tired.

The orthopaedic consultant saw me the day after I arrived home from France. He said he would send a physiotherapist to me the following morning to get me out of bed. I told him that would not be possible since I had been informed by my surgeon in France that I would not be sitting for another two weeks, let alone standing. The consultant was astonished that I was challenging him and asked me if I was refusing to be treated.

'No,' I said, 'I'm not refusing.' I was simply following the instructions of the doctors who had looked after me for the past five weeks. I told him that until my patient chart was available for him to read in English, I would not be going against the advice of the team in France. The consultant turned on his heel and left the ward.

Not long after this encounter, the staff nurse on the ward came in and admonished me for speaking to the consultant in such a way.

'What way?' I asked. I repeated what I had told him and said that I would cooperate fully once they had a chance to read the reports from my doctors in France.

The following morning, despite my protests, the physiotherapist appeared at my bed. I was furious. I told him there had been a mix-up and sent him on his way. The staff nurse dutifully reported back to the consultant that I had refused treatment.

This went on for a few days until the consultant decided to summon my parents. They made an appointment to see him and had to queue at one of his public clinics. He proceeded to tell them that I had an attitude problem and he asked them to have a word with me.

My mother decided instead that she would have a word with *him*. She told him that I was an adult and that I made my own decisions and that she agreed with my decision not to cooperate with the physiotherapist because it was against the advice I had received. And with that she stood up and motioned to my father to follow her. Dad, taken aback, promptly rose to his feet and they both walked out. When my patient chart was translated, there was no further talk of getting me out of bed, but there was no apology either. Case closed.

A week later, I was ready to sit up in the bed. The nurses propped the pillows up behind me as the physiotherapist helped me into a sitting position. My leg was suspended in the air on a loop dangling from the ceiling as it was still broken but couldn't be put in a cast because the skin graft on my ankle was still healing. It was all very uncomfortable.

I was sitting up and feeling sorry for myself, when I heard a voice I instantly recognised: Susan. 'Well hello there, Vicky!' I turned to look at the doorway, and there she was with Maria, followed in tow by Bernard and Mark. The girls, my best friends since childhood, were more like sisters to me, and Bernard and Mark I knew from college. We'd all become very close over the years. It gave me such a lift to see them bounding in, with all their usual energy. I had missed them over the past few months.

Susan and Maria were trained nurses. They both asked questions about how I was healing and how I was feeling. They could tell my spirits were low.

'Would you not come outside for a bit of air?' Maria asked.

I gestured towards the wheelchair in the corner of the room. 'It would have to be on that awful thing,' I said.

It was the kind of chair you don't see anymore, with the padding all the way up to the crown of your head, meant for geriatrics.

'Sure let's give it a go!' said Susan, seeing me perk up at the idea of doing something a bit different.

'I haven't been outside in months,' I said nervously.

'All the more reason!' said Maria. 'It's a beautiful day out there.'

Bernard moved the wheelchair into position and Mark checked that the coast was clear.

I must be out of my mind, I thought, to let them do this.

Mark and Bernard carefully lifted me into the chair, with Susan and Maria giving instructions. They propped pillows under my leg to keep it outstretched.

'Let's get out of here!' whispered Maria.

They pushed me out of the room, and zoomed down the narrow corridor. We gathered speed as they propelled me out the double doors of the entrance to the hospital and into the fresh air. 'Wahoooo,' they yelled. 'Shawshank style!'

They continued running and pushing the wheelchair. We were all laughing and cheering. It was the first time I had laughed in a long time. People were looking out their car windows. A man passing by stopped to ask if we were doing a run for charity. We laughed so hard we had to stop to catch our breath.

'Do you fancy a pint?' Susan suggested, with a cheeky grin on her face.

'What?' I said. 'You've got to be joking!'

'You're grand sure, we're both nurses,' said Maria, with a wink. 'We'll prescribe a pint of cider!'

'It's just the day for it,' said Susan. And it really was a summer cider kind of day.

Before I knew it they had snuck me down the road and into the car park of The Cove pub. Bernard disappeared for a minute, and then re-emerged with one of the barmen, opening the emergency exit at the back of the pub to get the wheelchair in the door.

They pushed me in and propped me up against the bar. I can't imagine what I must have looked like, with my suspended leg and my scars and bandages. But I didn't care. It was the most normal I'd felt in a long time.

'Cheers!' said Susan as we all clinked glasses.

I only managed a few sips. 'We'd better get back,' I said. 'They'll kill us if they find out.'

They pushed me back up the road and into the grounds of the hospital. We all tried to look a little more sombre so as not to draw attention to ourselves. It wasn't easy though, as we still had the giggles. As we came in through the hospital entrance, who was standing there only my mother. Her arms were crossed, and if looks could kill, well, hers would have. We're in for it now, I thought.

'How could you!' she scolded. 'And the two of you are nurses! You should know better.'

Bernard and Mark quietly pushed me back into the ward, while Maria and Susan stayed to face the wrath. We still laugh now, though, thinking back on that day. Our very own *Shawshank Redemption*!

*

Another few weeks went by and the doctors decided it was time I tried to walk. It was a strange concept, having to learn that basic skill again. When I was a one-year-old I learned to walk, with my mother's hands holding mine, back in our little cottage in Kilkenny. The first of many steps to come, safe in my mother's care. As long as I kept moving forward, no matter how unstable I was on my feet, she would be there to catch my fall.

And now, here I was, at the age of nineteen learning to do it all again. This time I had to learn to do it myself. I put my foot on the ground, carefully, and immediately an excruciating pain shot up through my leg. 'I can't do it,' I said, 'it's too painful.' I fell back onto the bed.

With some encouragement, I tried again, but the same thing happened. Then I tried a third time, and a fourth, until eventually I was standing. I looked at the physiotherapists in disbelief.

'You're doing it!' they said, coaxing me.

I cried with relief. I had wondered if I would ever walk again. I started off slowly, standing with the help of a Zimmer frame. The physiotherapists were encouraging me. 'Just one step,' they said. 'You can do it. Nice and slow.' I was exhausted.

We went through the same routine day after day. But as time wore on, I was becoming disheartened at the lack of progress. The physios said I was coming on, but I couldn't see it. Incremental progress, they told me. I was getting there.

And they were right. I soon graduated to crutches once I was steady on my feet. They were difficult to master. My ribs hurt, as did my collarbone, and I was getting welts on my hands from leaning on them. My legs felt as heavy as sandbags, as if they were not my own. There were days when I couldn't deal with the pain. I stayed in bed, not moving.

Until one day I finally did it. I stood up and slowly, agonisingly, placed one foot in front of the other. Tears were rolling down my cheeks. I needed to sit down again. That was enough for one day, they decided. My first step. The first of many more to come.

This routine continued day after day, until finally, with the help of two physiotherapists, one either side of me, I managed to walk five steps. It was the closest I had come to walking in months. I was tired and out of breath and needed to rest. I was relieved. I could see light at the end of the tunnel. Maybe one day I would walk properly again.

I thought of Katy. She was paralysed for life. Just a couple of months ago we were sitting in the same car, only in different seats. Now here I was, learning to walk again. She would never know that feeling; the rest of her life would be spent in a wheelchair. I knew I was very lucky to have survived, and to be getting back to myself again.

A few weeks later I was moving around on my own, shuffling to the end of the ward and back. A little independence at last. After what felt like a long time, they were finally ready to discharge me. I had spent the best part of three months in hospital. Home for plenty of rest, is what they prescribed.

But I had other plans, and I announced to my parents that I was going back to college. It was mid-October, the term had already started, and I was determined not to miss any more. 'I can move on my own now,' I told them indignantly as I hobbled around, quite unconvincingly.

The doctors and my parents were adamant that I was not yet ready for college, and that the best thing would be to take a year out. But the thought of not completing my college course, having worked so hard to get there, was something I was not prepared to entertain. This is what happens to people, I thought. I'll intend to take a year out, and then I'll never go back. It will be something I'll always regret. My life will take on some other trajectory, working a local job, or settling down with someone. I wasn't about to let that happen.

I continued to argue my point, telling my parents I was old enough to make my own decisions. And with that, I found myself back on the UL campus, crutches in hand. I had forgotten how far from one another each of the lecture halls was. Or perhaps I'd never noticed when I was in my full health. But now, I could feel every agonising step. People who knew me looked on in sympathy as I tried to navigate my way from one lecture to the next. It was exhausting.

After three weeks, I had to give in. It was all too much. I was in pain most of the time, and wasn't able to concentrate on my studies. Getting around the campus was too much for me. I had to concede and go home to rest.

11

A Birthday To Remember

THEY HAD THE SITTING ROOM set up for me, with the sofa propped up with pillows, so I would have somewhere to rest during the day. In a way it was comforting being back in my parents' house, though part of me felt like I was regressing, being back in the cradle of their care. I had only recently found my wings. Like the starling at the window, I had flown off into the night, only to find myself back again, tethered and broken.

As the weeks wore on, I was becoming more and more introverted. Hospital had made me afraid of things and my attempt at going back to college had knocked my confidence. The whole experience had made my world very small.

'Would you not give Maria or Bernard a shout?' Mam would say.

'Ah, maybe another time,' I'd reply. I didn't have the energy and I found it difficult to talk to people. I didn't have much to say; there wasn't much happening in my life. I felt I had failed at going to college, and I couldn't bring myself to speak about

France, and no one dared to ask, as word had spread around the village of my terrible accident abroad.

But I was thinking about France all the time. In my mind I was walking through the streets of Péronne, hand in hand with Christophe, and listening to the jukebox late into the night. I wondered if I would ever be that person again, if I'd ever be the same. I didn't think I would be. I couldn't imagine feeling any of those feelings again: happiness, love. They all felt very foreign to me now.

There's a happiness in youth when you feel like nothing bad can or will ever happen. We don't appreciate it until we've crossed over to the other side, where people know pain. And then you feel numb. It never really goes away; it's just a numb pain that's constantly there. I felt like I had crossed over. I was seeing people in a different way now, wondering what pain they knew, which side of the line they were on. I envied those who still lived in that way – not knowing the depth of what pain is. In some ways I resented them. I felt they would never really understand. They lived in a different world.

I was sleepwalking through life. Mam encouraged me to go on little outings. I went for lunch with her one day in town. Ronan, a guy I had kissed a few years ago, was there too sitting at a table across from us. I could see him looking over, trying to catch my eye. I looked down at the table and focused hard on the conversation with Mam so as not to draw his attention. I didn't have it in me to talk to him, never mind the thought of being with him. Or anybody else, for that matter. The idea of kissing someone or being intimate with them, anybody other than Christophe, made me feel sick. My body was shattered and my head and heart were hurting. I had never felt so low. I was carrying a heavy sadness with me everywhere I went.

That night as I undressed in my bedroom I looked at my naked body in the mirror. I was a broken thing. My broken wings. I ran my fingers over my scars. I couldn't imagine anyone looking at me and seeing anything but scars and broken limbs, and all the pins and stitches that were holding me together. Like a ragdoll.

The next morning I didn't get up when the alarm went off. Instead I stayed in bed. I put a CD on and listened to Tom Petty's 'Learning To Fly' on repeat from under the comfort of my duvet. Flashbacks of the crash were coming back to me. When I closed my eyes I could smell the burning flesh. The thought haunted me. I could feel the darkness, the blackness of nothing and the strong stench through the air.

It was a special day – 28 October 1994, my twentieth birthday. I lay there listening to the moving lyrics – about learning to fly – but having no wings, feeling empty.

I remembered all the times I had played the song in Péronne with Christophe.

I knew Mam and Dad would try to make a fuss. But it's not about the cake, is it, birthdays, I thought to myself. It's about celebrating that you've lived another year – that you were one of the lucky ones who made it through. I knew I was lucky. But I didn't feel lucky. I felt angry that Christophe would never see his nineteenth birthday. Or any birthday again. Why did I deserve it, if he didn't? I was struggling with the guilt of having survived. I felt like Christophe was the only one who would understand.

I took out my notepad and wrote him a letter. 'Dear Christophe …'

I wrote in French. It's how we always spoke to one another. I told him it was my birthday, that I had finally turned twenty. I told him all the things I wished I had said to him while he was still here. And I told him I was sorry. Sorry that I had lived. I told him how hard life was without him, and how much I missed him.

I signed the letter, 'With all my love, Vicky'.

There were so many things I hadn't said, so many things I wish I had said while I had the chance. Now all I could do was write letters that he would never read. Over the months I wrote to him many times over. Whenever I missed him and wanted to tell him something.

At other times in my life I would have prayed to God to make things better. I couldn't bring myself to pray now. I had started to blame God for what happened. I knew I shouldn't. But the same questions kept going through my mind: why did He let this happen to us? What did we ever do to deserve such a punishment? And where was Christophe now?

I turned on the CD player again. This time it was Dire Straits, *Brothers in Arms* one of Christophe's favourite songs. The opening verse played as I laid my head on the pillow. I closed my eyes and pretended Christophe was beside me as the melancholic lyrics filled the room.

12

Unfinished Business

THE WEEKS PASSED AND THE days seemed to have very little meaning anymore. When there's nowhere for you to go, Monday and Sunday are one and the same. There was no sense to things. I felt like I was living in a daze. Life revolved around little else other than mealtimes and sleep. Though spending time with Lyndsey always cheered me up. She would bound into the room with news from school or a new piece of gossip for me. Sisters are great like that. They're always there. Even when she was too young to really realise what that meant, she was still there for me, in her own way.

One morning, I was outside the house, leaning on my crutches. Mam had told me to get out for some air. A daily ritual. I did it to please her. I knew deep down it was good for me though, and I always felt better afterwards. It was a crisp winter day. My mind was lost in thought, when I looked up to see a funeral car pass by with a coffin inside. I went to cross myself, out of a lifelong learned habit – but then stopped. Sometimes I forgot that God and I were no longer friends. I hesitated a moment, then crossed myself out of respect for the dead. The person in the coffin probably believed in God and had crossed themselves all their life. It seemed only right. A gesture to send them on their way.

I wondered what Christophe's funeral had been like. It frightened me to think of it. To think of him being placed in the cold hard ground, covered in earth. Still. Motionless. Gone.

There's closure in ceremony. There's a reason we have ritual around death, I thought, as I stood watching the funeral procession passing. I had often heard it said that we do death well in Ireland. I'm not sure what that means, but I think it comes down to how we gather together as a community and how we process the loss of someone.

I hadn't been able to go to Christophe's funeral. There had been no closure. It felt as though he was always just in the next room, just out of reach, out of sight. I couldn't accept that he was gone.

I decided I needed to do something about it; I had unfinished business in France. I went back into the house to formulate a plan. I rang the Hotel Mercure. The international dial tone sounded eerie, like channelling into another world.

'*Bonjour*,' the voice answered. I recognised it as that of the receptionist.

'*Bonjour, Muriel. C'est moi, Vicky.*' There was silence for a moment as she processed what I had said.

'Vicky from Ireland?' she asked.

'Yes,' I said.

'It's good to hear from you, Vicky.' She sounded surprised. I'm sure the accident had sent shockwaves through the hotel.

I asked her for Christophe's home address and telephone

number. She was very helpful. She recited it to me and I scribbled it down. I ended the call and took out a piece of paper to write a letter to Christophe's parents.

It was hard to know what to say. It had been nearly six months since the accident and I hoped they were coping. I told them I was still on crutches, but recovering well. Missing Christophe all the time as I was sure they must be. And then I got to the nub of it. I asked how they would feel about me coming over to visit them in France. I told them that Christophe spoke of them often and that I would love to meet them and to visit his grave. If it was too soon for them I would understand and I could always come another time, when it suited them better.

I reread the letter and hesitated before putting it in the envelope. It was hard to know if I was imposing. I hoped they wouldn't see it that way.

Later that afternoon when Mam was going into town to do the grocery shop I asked her if she would post a letter for me.

'Of course,' she said.

I handed her the envelope. I saw her glance at the name and address as she put it into her bag. She recognised the name: Pellenz. She looked at me quizzically.

'I just want to see how they are,' I said.

I knew my mother wished I would leave France behind me. I was safe in Ireland now and the thought of France brought everything back to her, memories she was trying to block out. I could tell she was proud of me, though, for checking in. It was the kind of thing she had raised me to do.

Two weeks went by. Every day when the postman arrived I checked the mat inside the door, expectantly. I wondered if I would ever hear back. I hoped they hadn't taken my letter the wrong way, or felt I was intruding. As the days wore on I began to feel embarrassed to have asked them if I could visit. I was a complete stranger at what must have been the hardest time in their lives.

Then one day, a letter arrived. 'Vicky, post for you!' Mam called from the kitchen.

I hobbled in on my crutches and sat down at the kitchen table. The envelope had a French stamp. I opened it hurriedly. My mother watched me as I read the letter. After a few minutes I put it down and announced, 'I'm going back to France.'

I knew from Mam's expression that she was upset. I explained that I needed closure. 'I need to see Christophe's grave and talk to his parents,' I said.

I could see a sadness come over her, sad that I had gone through so much at such a young age, and a fear that I was putting myself in harm's way again. I hoped she wouldn't make me argue my case.

'It's just the thought of you being back in France. It frightens me.'

'I know. But I'm not going to be able to recover unless I do this. I need to do it,' I explained.

'You can barely walk,' Mam pleaded. 'Would you not wait a few more months – until you're a bit stronger?'

I looked at her, a look she knew well. This was something I was going to do. With or without her blessing.

Christophe's parents had said how much my letter meant to them, and how much they would love to have me stay. They asked me to call them to make the arrangements as soon as possible. I called them the next day.

As the foreign dial tone sounded, I suddenly felt nervous about what I would say or how the conversation would go.

A woman answered. '*Bonjour.*'

'*Madame Pellenz?*'

'Vicky?'

'Yes, it's me,' I said.

'Vicky, it's so good to hear from you. We've been waiting for your call.'

We talked for just a few minutes.

'Fly to Luxembourg. It's the nearest airport,' she said. 'We'll collect you.'

'Are you sure it suits you?' I asked.

I wanted to gauge how they felt about the whole thing.

'It would mean a lot to us, Vicky. We would love to see you.'

I thanked her and hung up.

The next day Mam gave me a lift into town. I went straight into the travel agency and booked the flights. Within a few days I had it all organised. I felt better than I had in a long time – it was like I had a place to focus my energy, something proactive I could do for Christophe.

When I arrived in Luxembourg airport I made my way slowly through the terminal on my crutches. I hadn't brought much luggage, just a small bag with a few essentials: a couple of changes of clothes and some gifts from Ireland for Christophe's family.

I stopped in the bathroom to check myself in the mirror. I looked different now. I didn't see myself in my reflection. My hair was short. I had lost a lot of hair after the accident through alopecia. Clumps had fallen out so I decided to cut it short. My nose was a different shape and my scars were still prominent on my face. I studied myself from head to toe, balancing on the crutches. A sore reminder for Christophe's parents of the accident and all that had happened. I wished I looked better. I put some makeup on and smoothed my hair. I wanted to make a good impression.

These were very different circumstances in which to meet your partner's parents. I wished Christophe was there, that we were going through arrivals together, to be greeted by happy hugs and introductions. That's the way I had imagined it. Instead, here I was, bruised and battered, and without Christophe.

I took a deep breath and headed for the arrivals hall. I saw them straight away: Christophe's parents, Bernadette and Christian, and his little sister, Mylène. She was only four years old, and was holding her mother's hand. She was beautiful, just like Christophe, with dark hair, sallow skin and brown eyes. I recognised them immediately. They all looked so like him. I waved over.

'Vicky?' they called.

'Yes!' I said.

'Welcome!' they said as we hugged one another. I quickly transitioned to French, as I knew they spoke very little English. They helped me with my suitcase and we made our way to the car park outside. Suddenly it dawned on me what I was doing. I wondered if it was all a bit strange – coming to meet the parents, when my boyfriend was dead – and if they were really okay with it. Perhaps they felt they couldn't say no. I hoped it wouldn't be an awkward few days. In the car I sat in the back with Mylène; she was so young and innocent. I wondered if she would remember her big brother at all when she was older.

His parents were full of conversation, asking about how I had been and how I was recovering. We didn't talk about Christophe. It was like we all had an unspoken understanding that that would come later, when we had all settled in.

The trip to the house took less than an hour. They brought

me into the dining room and introduced me to Christophe's younger brother, Gael, who was fifteen. He didn't know where to look or how to react when he saw me coming in on crutches. A sore reminder of his brother's accident.

They had been waiting for me to have dinner so Christophe's mother busied herself with getting the food ready, while I sat and chatted to his dad, who selected a nice bottle of wine for us to have with our meal. I looked around the house, trying not to look like I was looking. This was where Christophe had grown up, where he had eaten his meals. I thought of all the family dinners he must have had at this very table, as I sat down in what I suspected was his seat.

I wondered what he would have thought of the situation, if he would have done the same thing had the roles been reversed. Would he be sitting at our kitchen table in Mooncoin, with the same thoughts?

Bernadette placed a speciality of the region in front of me, a quiche Lorraine, which she had cooked especially for me, along with a salad. 'Please, help yourself,' she said, smiling. 'Is this okay for you?' I could tell she was nervous, trying to make sure I was well looked after.

When we were all settled around the table, she turned to me. 'Vicky, we'd like to hear more about Christophe ... how was he in Péronne? We have heard so little about what happened.'

'Not now,' Christian said, shooting her a stern look. 'She has just arrived.'

They locked eyes for a moment. I could see Bernadette was anxious for news.

'Sorry, Vicky,' she said, after a moment. 'It's just been very hard.'

I suddenly felt the weight of what I represented to them. Of what I was there to do. I was the last person who had seen their son alive. 'He was very happy in Péronne,' I said. 'Very happy. And he was such a great worker, and everybody loved him. They really did.' I could feel the tears welling in my eyes as his mother looked at me, taking in every word.

'Thank you, Vicky.'

'Maybe we can talk some more tomorrow,' suggested Christian, trying to manage the situation. He must have experienced a lot of emotional evenings in the past few months, I thought.

Christian quickly changed the subject. We talked of Beuvange, the little village where they lived, and of Mooncoin, and Ireland, which they had never visited. It felt false in a way to talk of frivolous things, when something so important was happening, but it's what we all needed to get through the evening.

Bernadette produced a cheese board and another bottle of wine. I asked about their lives and where they were from and how they met, even though I knew a lot about them already from conversations with Christophe. I knew that they had met when they were teenagers, just like my parents. In a way, I think Christophe and I bonded over that similarity. When we spoke about it in Péronne, in the back of our minds we both imagined that the same thing might happen to us – that we might end up together, having met as teenagers.

'Would you be okay staying in Christophe's room?' Bernadette asked as they began to clear the table.

'Pardon?' I said, unsure that I had heard her correctly.

Christian took over. 'We're wondering if you would feel alright about sleeping in Christophe's room. It's just that we don't have a spare room ...'

I hesitated. I hadn't expected this. 'Well, more importantly, how do you feel about that?' I said. 'I would be very happy to sleep on the couch.'

'No, Vicky, you are still recovering,' said Bernadette. 'Christophe would have liked you to stay in his room. I'll show you where it is and you can settle in.'

She stood up from the table. I took hold of my crutches and followed her down the hallway.

'Just here,' she said, reaching into the room and turning on the light.

I stood in the doorway, leaning on my crutches. There were posters on the walls around his neatly made bed. A vase of flowers stood on the bedside locker. They seemed somewhat out of place – a feminine touch in what was otherwise a very masculine teenage boy's room. Put there especially for me, I thought. I looked at Christophe's mother. I could only imagine how hard this must be for her. How much she was trying to welcome me, despite her own emotions.

'Thank you,' I said. 'It's lovely.'

'Just as he left it,' she said wistfully.

We said goodnight. I closed the door and sat on the bed. Just as Christophe must have done many times throughout his life, I thought. It was strange to be there, surrounded by so many pieces of Christophe – but without him.

There were posters on the walls of bands he liked and photographs of him and his friends blu-tacked to the headrest of the bed. In every photo he seemed to be laughing and smiling in the sun. It was nice to see him happy, to see what his life was like outside of Péronne. A happy life filled with people.

I looked through the CDs on his desk – all his favourites: Tom Petty, Dire Straits, Pink Floyd. All the songs he used to play on the jukebox in Péronne. I sat at his desk. There were notes scribbled on Post-its and notebooks – things he was thinking about. What happens to the thoughts, I wondered, when our brains are no longer active? Where do they go? All the things we imagine, all the thoughts and ideas that make us who we are. Suddenly gone.

I closed my eyes and tried to hear his voice. It was hard. I felt like I could feel the outline of him but already there were missing parts. I felt such a deep sadness for his parents. They had lost a huge part of their lives – such a bright, wonderful boy. But not only that, they had lost everything he would become and the family he may have had one day. When someone is killed, all the people that would have come after them are also killed. He would have been a great dad, I thought, looking at photos of Christophe with his little sister.

It's amazing, really, I thought to myself, all the people through time who had to stay alive long enough to make you, you. The tiny possibility of that is incredible. We are so lucky to be given a chance at life at all. But to cut a life off so soon, there can be no reason in that.

Everything seemed very surreal. I still felt like he would walk into the room at any moment, as though I was visiting his parents with him, which should have been the case. I opened the wardrobe and pressed his clothes against my face, taking in the familiar scent of him. I fell asleep clutching his shirt to my chest. A shirt without the body that used to be inside it: no chest to lay my head on and listen to his pounding heart, no arms to hold me through the night.

The next morning I woke to the smell of coffee. For a moment I thought I was back home. I got a fright when I sat up to see a photo of Christophe beside the bed, but then I remembered where I was.

I quickly got dressed and made my way to the kitchen. It was full of the noise of family life. Christophe's sister was sitting at the table, colouring. I wondered if she understood all that had happened, if she knew her big brother was never coming back.

'Morning,' I said, trying to keep the tone light.

'Ah, good morning, Vicky!' said Christophe's father, pouring me a coffee and signalling for me to join him at the table.

As the day wore on, his mother was full of questions for me. I could see his parents were clinging to any part of him that they could reach and I was the closest they had come in a long time. His mother was very maternal. Her eyes reminded me of Christophe's eyes. Sometimes it was hard to look at her because she was so like him.

Christophe's grandmother lived next door. They had told her I was visiting and suggested I go and say hello. Her eyes lit up when she saw me and she had a warm smile. 'You must be Vicky,' she said. 'Come in, please.'

When I stepped inside she gave me a long hug, the kind you give a child who's upset. It was comforting. She welcomed me into her kitchen. Her house was small and filled with trinkets. She had a statue of Jesus and the Sacred Heart on the wall, which reminded me of my own grandmother's house. As we sat over a cup of coffee and a pastry at the kitchen table, she showed me her miraculous medals and told me stories about when Christophe was young. I could see she loved him very much. I was glad she had religion, to help her through.

'Do you pray?' she asked me.

I hesitated for a moment. 'I used to,' I said.

'I pray,' she said. 'It helps.'

That evening over dinner, Christophe's parents asked if I would like to visit his grave the next morning. It was a big part of why I had come, but now that I was here, the reality was almost too much to take in.

In the morning we walked to the cemetery, his mother chatting to me all the while. I tried to follow the conversation, but found it hard to concentrate; I was trying to mentally prepare myself for seeing Christophe's headstone. His father was quiet. I couldn't imagine how hard it was for them. The last time they saw their child he was fit and healthy and full of life. Then, from nowhere, there was a knock on their door: a policeman come to say he had died. How could the human brain fathom that? I wondered. Some things are just too much.

We arrived at the graveyard and walked slowly and quietly through the rows of headstones. I read the names as we passed, the names of old people – grandparents, mothers, fathers – and young people – sons and daughters, sisters and brothers. Their birth date and their dying day carved forever in stone, their lives in between, everything they were and everything they did. The beginning, the middle and the end.

And then I saw it: Christophe Pellenz. Born 6 September 1975 – Died 10 July 1994. I looked at that second date. It was etched in my consciousness. I could remember every minute of that day.

Everything flashed through my mind – the decision to go to the club, getting into the car, Christophe at the wheel. Every part of me wished I could go back in time and tell him not to get into the car. All the 'what ifs' kept playing on a reel: what if we hadn't gone out, what if we had just gone to our usual place in Péronne, what if it had been me instead of him? Christophe would still be alive, not six feet under the cold, hard ground. I was the last person to see him alive. I still had the image of him in my mind, sitting beside me in the car.

Christophe's mother took a tissue from her coat pocket. Her husband put his arm around her as she cried against his chest.

I placed the flowers beside the headstone. I wanted to cry but I couldn't. I felt like I was in a dream, that none of it was real, like I was outside of myself, watching the scene rather than being a part of it. And yet when I looked at Christophe's parents, and saw the pain in their eyes, my chest felt heavy. I wanted to say something to them, to comfort them, but I didn't have the words. His mum gave me a hug. She held me tight as she cried. It was then that I started to cry as I felt her breaking down against my body. I could feel her giving in to the pain. We both gave in to it. I couldn't imagine what she must be feeling, to lose a son, her baby, at the age of eighteen. A child.

The walk home was silent, each of us lost in our own minds and memories. Trying to come to terms. When we got back to the house, Christophe's mum smiled at me as she gathered herself. 'Cup of coffee?' she asked.

'That would be nice,' I said.

There was something cathartic about having expressed our emotions to one another. I felt closer to her now, more connected.

I could see they liked having some adult company around the house. Christophe's sister was being minded by her grandmother for the afternoon and Gael was at school. As we sat down, I asked if they had seen many of Christophe's friends since the accident.

'Not really,' Christophe's father said. 'They are teenagers. They find it hard to know what to say to us.'

I looked around the house. I knew from Christophe's stories

of home that it had once been a noisy place full of friends visiting for sleepovers. The silence must be very hard for them, I thought as I looked at the framed photograph of Christophe on the dresser. He was smiling that incredible smile of his, so full of life. A moment frozen in time.

'There was one day …' said Bernadette '… I went to the grave to change the flowers. I saw Christophe's best friend Samuel there. I was so happy to see him. It felt like getting a part of Christophe's life back, even just for a few minutes. When I got closer I saw that he was crying. "Hi Samuel," I said. He looked up and as I approached I could see he was embarrassed to be upset. He didn't know where to look or what to say to me. But he didn't have to say anything. He didn't need the right words. I just wanted to give him a hug.'

I nodded. 'It's hard to know what to say,' I said.

'He was awkward and rushed away quickly,' she continued. 'I asked him to come to see us at the house. He used to be in our house all the time. We missed seeing him. But he never came again.' Her voice trailed off as she stared out the window, lost in memories.

'I can understand,' said Christian. 'They are teenagers and it's very emotional. Before you arrived, Vicky, it was like he never existed. He had just vanished, and every part of his life was gone.'

'I'm glad I came,' I said. 'It was the same for me. Nobody at home knew Christophe. Seeing you has helped me too.'

'Well, you meant a lot to him,' said Bernadette. 'He told us all about you and he was delighted he had an Irish girlfriend.'

'He said he planned to go to Ireland someday,' his father added.

'I wish he had,' I said. 'He would have loved it. My parents are very like you. And my home is very like your home.'

They smiled at the thought. I told them how Christophe and I had often talked about how similar our families were. Both our mums loved to knit. Our dads were great with their hands. And we both came from happy homes.

A few days later, it was time for me to go. It was hard to say goodbye, but I promised to stay in touch and to come back again soon. We had all healed a little from our time together. It had been good for all of us. And now, real life was about to resume again. Me in Ireland, and them piecing together a new life without their son, the best way they could.

As I headed off in the taxi I looked back as they waved goodbye from the doorstep. I waved too, until they disappeared into the distance. I felt like I was leaving a world that could have been a second home to me. If Christophe had survived, and we had ended up together, this place would have been a big part of our lives. I imagined going to meet his parents for the first time together, then later as a more established couple for visits, then maybe in time, with our own children. They could have been my children's grandparents. My parents-in-law. But it was not to be.

13

Some Things Should Never Go Unsaid

THERE WAS SOMETHING ELSE I needed to do before I left France, something I hadn't told anyone about.

In the hospital they told me about how we were saved the night of the accident. My mother had cut out newspaper clippings from the local French newspapers when she was there. She knew that I would want to see the photos of the crash and to read what had been reported in the media. As well as the photos of the two cars, there was information about the man who had pulled us from the wreckage, a fireman named Eddie Dekydtspotter. He was awarded a medal for his bravery. He was off-duty that night when he saved three lives. We would all have died had he not pulled us from the burning car. I tried to imagine what it must have been like for him, to run towards danger like that, putting himself in harm's way to save our lives.

I took the train bound for Péronne. It would be difficult to be back there, but this was something I needed to do. After a long journey, I made my way towards the house I was looking for.

Standing on a quiet suburban street, I took the crumpled note out of my jeans pocket to check the address they had given me at the fire station.

This was his house, the man who saved my life. It was a small traditional French dwelling with jaded paintwork and old-fashioned shutters on the windows. I knocked on the door and waited. Suddenly nervous.

The door opened and a plump elderly woman appeared. 'Welcome, welcome!' she said, kissing me on both cheeks and embracing me, pressing me against her chest. Before I knew what was happening she had hooked her elbow into mine and was helping me to navigate the stone steps with my crutches.

'Thank you,' I said. She gave me a smile. Her sea green eyes had a twinkle. It was hard not to be happy to meet her, but she wasn't who I was expecting. I was expecting a man. I wondered for a moment if I had the right house.

Once inside, she disappeared into the kitchen, gesturing for me to follow her. The house was dark and cool. I could see it was a home without much money to speak of, but that it was cared for and loved – everything neatly occupying its own special place. A wooden dresser stood in the kitchen. Beside it was an old cooker, which had a look of being much used. In the middle of the room was a carefully laid wooden table with a handmade crochet tablecloth draped over it and a vase filled with wildflowers. The kettle was whistling from the stove and the smell of freshly baked croissants filled the air. She opened the oven, and placed the baking tray on the counter for the croissants to cool. They looked hot and buttery and smelled very inviting. My stomach lurched with a sudden feeling of hunger.

I was about to tell her who I was, and ask if a Monsieur

Dekydtspotter lived in the house. I wanted to clear up any confusion, in case she had been expecting someone else. Though I sincerely hoped the croissants were intended for me as my mouth was watering with the smell of them.

Just as I went to say something, a man appeared in the frame of the door. '*Monsieur Dekydtspotter?*' I asked hopefully.

'Yes,' he said, taking his gloves off and wiping a bead of sweat from his brow. He looked to have just come in from the garden. There were grass stains on his clothes. 'But please, call me Eddie.'

'I'm Vicky,' I said, 'from the car accident at Fricourt. Thank you for agreeing to see me.'

Something flashed across his face. It happened so quickly I couldn't tell what it was. Perhaps for a moment he found himself back at the site of the crash.

'I just wanted to say thank you,' I said. He looked embarrassed.

'No, no need for thank you,' he replied, looking down at his feet. 'You have met my mother,' he said, gesturing towards the plump elderly lady.

She was pouring coffee into a shiny silver pot. It looked like something that was only used for special occasions. She looked at us both, and on her way back to the stove she planted a kiss on each of her son's cheeks. She was very proud of him, I could see that.

'She is very happy you have come,' he said.

I got the feeling he could have done without plaudits. He seemed humble. Unused to thanks or ceremony. 'Please sit down,' he said, moving towards the sink to wash his hands. I saw him glance at my crutches and down at my ankle as he passed.

'I'm healing very well,' I said, 'thanks to you.' They had told me in the hospital that, in order to save my life, he had to pull me from the debris, and my ankle was stuck beneath the twisted metal of the car. He knew it was only a matter of minutes before flames would engulf the car. He pulled hard, breaking my ankle, but saving my life.

Eddie said very little through the whole encounter. His mother asked me how I was feeling and if I was back living in Péronne. 'No,' I said, 'I live in Ireland. I just came back to visit.' I didn't go into the detail of seeing Christophe's family. I thought it may be too much for him to think of the dead boy's body, as he had found it in the car. I could only imagine the memories he carried with him from that night.

As we neared the end of our coffees, I felt it was nearly time to go. I looked him straight in the eye and said, 'Thank you … for saving my life.'

He looked bashfully down at his feet, not knowing what to say. I could see it meant a lot to his mother. It meant a great deal to me too. I owed my life to this man, a perfect stranger.

I gathered myself together and made my way back out into the summer sun. I said my goodbyes at the door and headed off down the laneway to meet my taxi. I could hear children playing nearby. I smiled at the sound of their laughter. I closed my eyes for a moment and took a deep breath.

I walked away knowing I had done the right thing. Some things are too important to go unsaid, I thought. I had done what I had come to do.

14

Starting Over

I HAD A RENEWED ENERGY after my trip to France. It was time to get my life back on track. Being abroad again reminded me of what I loved about travelling. I needed to go somewhere that didn't end in tragedy, to prove to myself that the world wasn't such a scary place. If I didn't do it now, I was afraid my world would get very small and I would develop a fear of things.

I asked a college friend who was studying in Spain if she would put up a notice for me in her local town advertising an Irish au pair. Within a few days the ad was answered. A Spanish couple with two little girls were interested in having me come to work for them. I rang them and explained I had been in an accident and was still on crutches. I wondered if that might put them off. I reassured them that I was no longer on medication and had plenty of experience as an au pair. We hit it off and they seemed happy with the scenario. The next day I booked my tickets to Santiago de Compostela in the north of Spain.

My next call was to UL to see if they would allow me to attend classes at the university in Santiago de Compostela. They agreed to my request, so all that remained was to break the news to my parents.

I sat them down at the kitchen table. 'I have something to tell you,' I said, cautiously.

They listened apprehensively, wondering what could be coming next.

'I'm going to live abroad again,' I said.

My mother was furious. 'Vicky … it was one thing to go back to France. You've barely recovered. Look what happened the last time you went to live abroad.' She got up from the table and walked out of the room. I could tell she was upset.

My father turned to me. 'Why do you want to go, Vicky?' he asked.

'I have to prove it to myself, Dad, that I can do this without something bad happening. I'm worried I'll be scared of things otherwise.'

My father understood. He knew from fishing that if you had a bad experience on the water, you had to get back in the boat and not let your demons get to you. Besides, he could see that I was getting frustrated being at home. I was starting to argue with Mam more and more. I was hard to be around.

He tried to reassure my mother that it was the best thing for me to do, that being at home wasn't doing me any good. And so, at the beginning of February 1995, a year since I had left to work abroad in France, I was making my way to Spain, crutches in hand.

I spent five wonderful months in Spain au pairing and attending classes at the University of Santiago de Compostela, and making new friends. It was everything I hoped it would be. Getting back on the plane to Ireland, I felt I had achieved something. I had gone abroad, and not come back on a stretcher, and I had recovered physically from the accident. I was no longer on crutches and all my scars had healed up nicely. The world wasn't such a frightening place anymore.

A few weeks after I returned home from Spain, I had to go back to France to have an operation to remove the steel pin in my left thigh. My parents came with me for support. It was strange to be back in the hospital in Amiens.

It was my first time to see the hospital properly. I was unconscious when I was taken there by helicopter and I was on a stretcher when leaving it to go back to Ireland. My parents showed me around. It had become a second home to them during the time they spent there. They showed me the room I was in, the little shop where my mother used to go to buy her bottle of Orangina after she got dehydrated, the accommodation they stayed in. It helped me to understand what that time must have been like for them.

Some of the nurses remembered me. They were delighted to see me walking back in, and admitted me for the operation. Mam and Dad stayed with Katy's mother, Sarah, in Lille that night and returned to the hospital the following day. I was back on crutches again. I would be on them for eight weeks until my leg healed.

Dad helped me into the taxi. They were bringing me back to Katy's house. I suddenly felt apprehensive. It was the first time I would see Katy since the accident. We had been in contact a lot over the past year, writing letters and phoning one another, but seeing her would be different.

Sarah met us at the door. 'Vicky! We've been so looking forward to seeing you!'

I could see that Sarah had been a great support for my parents, and they for her. They had experienced something life-changing together. They understood what the other had gone through, in a way none of us could, not even me and Katy.

They brought me through to the living room. Katy was there, sitting in her wheelchair. At first it seemed normal to see her sitting there, as though she were sitting on the sofa. But then the reality sunk in when it was clear that she could not stand up. She was paralysed from the neck down. She'd had a tracheostomy, a procedure where an opening is surgically made through the neck to provide an airway so that the person can breathe. Katy had severed her spinal cord and was unable to breathe following the accident so she had to breathe this way, via a tube.

'Hi, Katy,' I said, smiling, trying to make it as normal as possible.

'Vicky,' she said. Her voice sounded very different. I could see she was struggling to speak, but her eyes lit up in the way that they used to.

I had a flashback to her dancing in the middle of the circle in the club that night. I moved to give her a hug. Her mother reminded me that she had no power in her arms. I hugged her anyway, as best I could.

She was so debilitated. Seeing it for myself made it all very real. She was able to control her electric wheelchair, but there was very little else she was able to do. I stayed with Katy and her family for two weeks.

Nurses came to the house every day to feed and wash Katy and to help care for her. It was heart-breaking for me to see her like that but I tried to be positive and to remind myself that she was still the same person that I knew when we shared the room in Péronne and that I was there to spend time with her and to be her friend.

We talked about the accident and what we remembered of that night. It felt like a dream, as if it were someone else's life we were remembering. We talked about Christophe and Lisa. Katy asked me what Christophe's parents were like and how they were doing. I put a CD on and we listened to some of the music we listened to in Péronne. It helped to bring us back to that time. It felt good to be normal with one another, to just be teenagers with each other again. We drank wine and stayed up talking at night, giving out about our mothers who were always fussing over us.

Soon it was time for me to go. We promised to keep in touch and made plans for Katy to come to visit Ireland when her condition became more stable.

Part of me felt guilty that my life could continue as it had been, when Katy's could not. I was getting ready to start college again. It would be like pressing the refresh button, one year on since the accident. I was worried about going back a year behind everyone I had started college with, but the five months in Spain and the trip to France had given me new confidence. I could join in as people talked about their semesters abroad. But I needed my own space too, now more than ever before. I had received a small sum of money as part of the settlement from the car crash. I used it to rent a bedsit on my own. It meant I could study more and didn't have to worry too much about socialising with people.

For some reason, I started to distance myself from those I had known in college before the crash. It probably wasn't fair on them, but I couldn't keep up with the pace and I wasn't interested in partying or drinking. I found it easier to make new friends in my year, people I didn't have to explain the accident to and who had no preconceived idea of who I was. Because I wasn't who I used to be. I was a different person now. I became very serious after the crash. I felt changed. Not just physically, but every part of me felt different. I was less carefree, because I knew how bad things could get. I was anxious most of the time. I felt bitter too. I don't know how else to describe it. I felt like no one else understood because they didn't know what it was like to have survived an accident that had killed two people, two incredible people, who were there one minute laughing and joking and the next minute they were gone. Just like that.

I found ways of coping. I took up lifesaving. Swimming was good exercise as my bones and muscles were still rehabilitating. But it was more than that, something about meeting the fireman in France had taught me the importance of being equipped to save a life. And even though I was learning to save other people, it was swimming that saved me. I swam every day after college. Being in the water made me feel liberated and safe at the same time. There were no expectations, no limitations; just me and the water. I had time to think. Headspace away from the noise of life.

I also decided to learn how to drive. I had become very fearful about getting into cars with anyone except my dad and a few trusted people. My New Year's resolution for 1996 was to apply for and pass my driving test. I used the rest of the money I was given out of the settlement from the accident to buy my first car – a metallic-green Peugeot.

The first lesson didn't go well. The car stalled and I cranked the gears and burned the clutch, careening around corners and stopping abruptly. It was harder than I'd anticipated.

'It's like this for everyone for their first couple of times,' the driving instructor reassured me, seeing the frustration on my face.

I could see him eyeing up my scars. 'I was in a car crash,' I told him, frankly.

He shuffled in his seat and seemed to have a new focus on teaching me to drive well. A few months and a lot of lessons later, I was finally getting the hang of it. I sat the test and passed.

From then on I became the designated driver for all my friends. I had decided to give up drinking alcohol for a while. It was another thing that made me anxious. I hated being out of control.

It was around this time that I met Jim. I thought I'd never find love again after Christophe. But I did, and when I least expected it. Sometimes people just fall into one another. I've seen movies and read books about love that's all-encompassing, a passion that grows and leads to a fairy tale proposal. It wasn't like that for me and Jim. But it was love all the same. Just not from the get-go.

Typical of an Irish scenario, we met through mutual connections. At the time, Jim's sister Ciara was going out with my brother Robbie. They had been together for nine years. I had seen Jim in passing in the street, or in the pub, but the first time I properly met him, apart from just saying hello, was when I gave him a lift home.

It was Paddy's Night 1996 and the pub was packed, with everyone joining in the revelry. I still wasn't drinking so I had offered Robbie and Ciara a lift home, back to Ciara's parents' house, which was also, of course, Jim's house. When we were leaving the pub I felt a tap on my shoulder. I turned around and it was Jim. 'Mind if I come too?'

The four of us walked out to the car. Jim remarked on how much I looked like Robbie. 'You're the spit of him! You might as well be the same person,' he said.

I didn't react. I was wearing a denim shirt and white t-shirt and a pair of jeans. My hair was still really short. I had cut it into a short choppy style, because clumps were still falling out in the shower. I was also very skinny at the time.

I resembled my brother Robbie normally, but with the short hair I knew I looked even more like him. I was feeling self-conscious and Jim's comments had hit a nerve. I decided he was obnoxious.

It was his way of flirting. He tried again, goading me for some sort of reaction. 'Love the little green snot!' he said as he got into the car, insulting my Peugeot. Still I didn't react. He was infuriating.

When we arrived at the Phelans' house, Ciara and Robbie jumped out first. 'Would you not come in for a while?' asked Jim from the back seat.

Ciara and Robbie chimed in. 'Yeah, come on, Vicky!'

After some persuasion, I finally gave in. I parked the car and the four of us went into the house. Ciara motioned for us to be quiet as her parents were sleeping. We tip-toed up the stairs to what they called 'the music room'.

We got talking. Jim was passionate about music and seemed to know a lot about it. Something we had in common. Somewhere between talking about Kurt Cobain and The Stunning, I realised I was laughing. He had a good sense of humour and was easy to talk to. Maybe he's not so bad, I thought. He's a bit different. There was something about him I was attracted to. He could sense it, and seized his moment. He leaned over and gave me a kiss.

I thought no more of it after that. A kiss, that's all it was. But to Jim, it was something much more. After that night, he sent messages to me through my brother. 'Jim says hi,' Robbie would say, coming back from Phelans'.

'Tell him I'm busy,' I retorted.

Robbie raised his eyebrows and shrugged, 'Whatever.'

I couldn't understand why Jim was so interested in me. I didn't feel like the same person I used to be: flirty and fun. I was serious now and looked like a boy. What could he possibly want from me?

Eventually I squared up to him one night when we were in the pub. 'Look, I'm off to Limerick tomorrow and I'm not going to be back home until the end of May, until all my exams are done,' I said, assertively. I thought that would be enough to fend him off.

Back in Limerick I soon became engrossed in my studies again. I had very little time to think about home, let alone Jim. I spent my time swimming and studying.

When I visited my parents at the weekends, Jim was always in touch. We bumped into each other again in the pub. It was awkward. When we talked there was a tension there – as if there was something happening beneath the surface that neither of us was acknowledging.

When I finished my exams, I knew it was time to decide whether Jim and I had a future together. I needed to draw a line under things, once and for all. It seemed only fair. I agreed to go on a date with him. We went to the pub for a drink. Conversation was easy – we knew most of the same people.

There was always a lot to talk about. One date led to two, and before I knew it we had spent most of the summer together.

As the summer drew to a close, I was getting ready to go back to college. Jim suggested we go away together first. Somewhere warm, maybe? It was a big move, but I thought it might be nice to get away from Ireland for a while before term started. We booked a last-minute holiday to the Greek island of Kos, and spent two weeks there. We hired a scooter and explored the island and I introduced Jim to scuba diving.

When the holiday was over, we arrived into Dublin airport. I collected my luggage, he collected his. It symbolised our separate lives. The summer was over and it was time for me to go back to my studies, back to 'real' life, for the final push, my final year.

I could tell Jim found it hard to say goodbye this time. We had become used to being around one another. But I was glad of the excuse to go. I wasn't ready to settle down and I could feel myself starting to fall for him. I needed to get away.

The first semester would be spent abroad. That would give me time and space, I thought, to let things breathe. I was going back to Spain. The university arranged a work placement teaching English in a private school and off I went to a small town called Ciudad Real, about an hour south of Madrid. I lived in an apartment with three other girls from UL: Mary, Hilda and Rian. From the moment we arrived, we enjoyed the Spanish way of life and the freedom of being in a foreign country. We were meeting new people, having new experiences. I called home every few days from the local payphone.

One day I went to the phone armed with coins; I called my parents and we caught up on what was happening in Spain, and in Kilkenny. I hung up and looked down at the coins in my hand. I had enough to make another call. I dialled Jim's number.

To my surprise he told me he'd managed to get some time off work and he would be joining me for a month in Spain. 'Like we talked about,' he said. We had mentioned that he might try to come and visit, but I never thought it would actually happen.

'What will I do with him for a whole month?' I said to the other girls, when I was back in the apartment. A few days later, Jim arrived. It was strange at first, to see him there in Spain, in this new world I had carved out for myself. But soon it started to feel normal, in fact more than normal; it was nice. I liked having him there with me. And needless to say, we found things to do. We spent a lot of time in bed, and things were fiery and passionate between us, in a way that they hadn't been at home. Maybe it was the thrill of being in a different country, in a new environment.

When my time in Spain came to an end, I found myself back in UL for my final semester. Life had returned to normal. I was in the library again and the pressure was on to finish my final-year thesis and pass my exams. I didn't see much of Jim during this semester. I rarely went home to visit and I phoned him less and less. I felt guilty about it in a way, but I felt my studies needed to come first. And eventually, all the studying did pay off, when I received a first-class honours degree and an award for my thesis.

To my surprise, my thesis supervisor, Professor Angela Chambers, suggested I apply for a PhD. At first it seemed like a notional idea, but the more I thought about it, the more I wanted to do it. With her encouragement, I sent in the application. I waited for weeks, until one day I received a letter in the post. I tore open the envelope and read the opening lines: 'Dear Vicky, we are delighted to inform you ...'

It was good news. I had been awarded a scholarship. This

was the stepping stone I needed. Something to focus on, I thought. I could continue my studies. The girl from down the pound was on her way to a doctorate. It gave my life direction; when everything else felt out of control, I had college, and I had my studies.

I told my family the news, and Jim and my brother Robbie and Ciara came up to visit me to celebrate. It was good to see Jim again; it had been a while since we'd seen one another. When I was with him, I realised I had missed him. It felt very natural to be together, the four of us.

There was something very loyal about Jim. He was dependable. I knew he had waited for me, and that he would wait for me. I just didn't feel ready for a proper relationship yet. There were things I still needed to get out of my system, energy I needed to burn. I was scared of a settled life where things would slow down. I was worried they'd slow until they stopped, and then my life would get small and parochial. There was still so much more of the world I needed to see.

'Now that you're finished your course, we might see more of each other ...' Jim said as we were walking home one night.

I hesitated. 'I think I might head off somewhere for a while,' I said.

He looked at me with an air of despondency as if to say: you're running away again. But I was restless and needed to run away. A few days later I booked flights to go to America on a J1 student visa for the summer.

Walking through the New York streets, I took a deep breath, and sighed with relief. This was about the furthest thing I could imagine to rural Ireland. It felt good to be on the road again. I spent the summer living in Queens. I managed to find a job working at a telemarketing company in the city, near Greenwich. It was definitely a world away.

I worked with a group of African-American women, all a good deal older than me.

Somehow I found myself in among their clique. They would spend half the day talking on the phone to their boyfriends and mothers, trying not to get caught by the supervisor. It was hard to get a word in with all the conversation flying around the lunch table every day, all the latest gossip and chat.

One day one of the women, the leader of the posse, confided in me that she was having trouble in her relationship. 'Things ain't goin' so well,' she told me as we sat over our lunchtime sandwiches.

In my innocence I didn't fully understand what that meant. I wasn't even sure how to read between the lines, so I didn't ask any more questions. Something about her made it clear that she would offer things up if and when she felt like it – we played on her terms. I'd never met anyone like her before. She seemed so strong and independent, like she could fight her own corner.

A few days later she came in looking very shook and one of the other women told me quietly what was happening. Her boyfriend was hitting her. People aren't always what you think they are and you never know what someone is going through. She seemed tough, but she was vulnerable too, like any of us. I sometimes wonder where she is now and how her life turned out. It seemed like a hard life.

And New York could be very hard on people. When you see a place as a tourist, life often doesn't seem real. It's all in technicolour when you're on holidays and the people you meet are almost like characters setting the scene. But when you work somewhere you get to see the real side of a city, underneath its skin. That's what I loved about working abroad. You were living in real life, in all its manifestations. And you could be whoever you wanted to be.

America was the land of opportunity, but I could see how easily you could fall between the cracks. Especially when society allowed it. New York was different from anywhere else I had lived. Walking through the city, I felt completely anonymous, like no one could see me, even though I could see them. There were characters I saw every day on my way to work, like the homeless man who sat on the corner, shouting at people walking by. I passed him by and wondered how he ended up on the streets. People tried to walk around him, to avoid getting too close to him. That's some mother's son, I thought to myself. He was carried in someone's womb, cared for in someone's arms. To someone, sometime, he was the world and the world was his oyster. And now, here he was, begging, living hand to mouth as people walked by, ignoring him. The American dream turned nightmare. The result of a system that failed to care for people.

It's funny how lives pass each other by, connecting for a moment and then going their own way. We were just passing through. We were the quintessential J1 students – living in each other's pockets in rundown apartments for little to no rent. I was working long shifts and then meeting up with friends afterwards. I even had a few visitors. Maria and another friend, Laura, came out for a week. I did all the touristy things with them. It was magic. I had regained my sense of self. I felt like I could have fun again. I loved living in a different place. The smells were different, the air was different. There was also an energy about New York, when it was going your way, that was electric.

After a long, hot summer, I returned home to start work on

my PhD and to figure out what kind of relationship I wanted with Jim, if he still wanted to make a go of it.

Jim was in touch as soon as he heard I was home and wanted to meet up. We went for a drink. It was good to see him again. In all the distraction of being away I hadn't really had much time to think of life in Ireland or of Jim. But now that I was home, I realised there was something about him I kept coming back to. He was kind. And different from any other man I'd known. He was always there. No matter how far I roamed, when I got back, he was home. I thought about the woman in New York and how alone she must have felt in an abusive relationship, with no safety net, no one to call home. It made me appreciate how much Jim cared for me.

However, there was something about our relationship that was bothering me. It felt off-balance, like things were mostly on my terms – when I was coming, when I was going. Jim never made me feel guilty about that. He let me be myself and do my own thing in the world. But things seemed a bit unequal. I was always in the driving seat.

At least that's what I thought until a few weeks later when, over a drink, he surprised me. 'I'm going to Australia for a while,' he said.

'What?' I replied, taken off-guard.

'With one of the lads. For a few months ...' he said, watching for a reaction.

'I'm delighted for you, Jim. I think it's great that you are going to see a bit of the world,' I said instinctively, pretending to be nonchalant about it. But the truth was I would miss him.

And sure enough, a few weeks later, he was gone. This time he was the one running away. He was away for five months and I was the one left waiting. I suppose it evened things out, in a way. I understood what it was like to wait for someone to come home. We were closer after that. And things felt steady. We fell into each other, into life together. And we had a lot of fun.

The years went by and life took on a rhythm of its own. In 1999, at the age of twenty-five, I got a job with an air charter company in Shannon airport. Jim was working as a carpenter on building sites. The airport work wasn't really what I wanted to do with my life, especially after studying in a different field. I kept an eye out for other opportunities and less than two years later, in September 2001, I got a job as manager of UL's European Exchange Programmes. It was perfect. After all my time abroad in college, I was well suited to the role. I was also working part-time on my PhD so being back in a university environment was stimulating. Life was busy and we were both doing well.

We were trying to think ahead and be clever with our finances, to make a solid plan for the future. Jim and I bought two houses in Limerick with a first-time buyer's grant. We spent our evenings after work painting and decorating them. We rented one out, which gave us a small monthly income. We lived in the other and rented one of the rooms to a student. It was a good set-up – sure to put us in good stead for the future. But it all felt a little transitory, living with a student, in a place neither of us called home.

I missed Kilkenny and being near my family. At the time Jim's father was renovating an old farmhouse in Mullinavat, just twenty minutes from Mooncoin. 'Will we go have a look?' Jim asked.

He knew how much I wanted to be back in Kilkenny. We drove out to have a look at the house. It was old but it had character and it was spacious, surrounded by fields and countryside. It was a world away from suburban life in Limerick. We looked at each other, and we knew: this was it. We decided to give it a go. We would put our DIY skills into action again. We had lots of ideas for ways to improve the house. It had the potential to be a beautiful home.

We met with the bank and organised the loan. We continued to rent out one of the houses in Limerick and sold the other to pay for the deposit. We made about forty thousand euro on the sale; this went straight into buying the new house in Kilkenny. We packed up our entire lives into boxes. I gave up my job in UL and we moved to Mullinavat, to begin the next chapter. Finally, I felt ready to settle down.

Mam and Dad arrived to help us unpack. Between the four of us, eating sandwiches and drinking numerous cups of tea, we made good progress. I could tell Mam and Dad were very excited at the prospect of having us so close by. We laughed as they told Jim stories about life in the Kelly household when I was growing up.

I unpacked the picture frames and trinkets and placed them carefully on the bookshelves – photographs, souvenirs from our travels together, the little things that slowly made the place feel like ours, that made it feel like home.

The plan was working and everything was coming together. But there was still one question hanging over us. Marriage.

Three years earlier, Jim had proposed to me and we had agreed to get married, but we'd never got around to making the plans, despite announcing our engagement that Christmas, sporting a lovely ring I'd found in an antique shop. Now it was time to do the deed.

Some girls dream of the big white dress and fairy tale

wedding. It just didn't appeal to me. We did things our own way. Our plan was to elope. Since I was no longer working full-time, I had time to organise things.

It suited Jim too. He was always the quiet type and never thought much of weddings. Instead of having a big wedding, we decided to use the money to go somewhere together and have a proper five-star holiday. 'We'll run away together this time,' he said.

I was sitting on the sofa at home, flicking through travel brochures looking for inspiration, when I landed on a two-page spread about Sri Lanka. The photos were of exotic beaches and vast jungle terrain. The article talked about the thrill of travelling the blue train that twists through the countryside cutting into the hills, past tea plantations and colonial-style railway stations. I dreamt about throwing my legs out the side of the carriage and watching the world go by like the carefree travellers I saw in the photographs. They were tanned from the sun and looked like they were fresh out of the warm sea. I could almost smell the ocean. It looked like nowhere I had ever been before. Jim was excited about it too. So we decided – we were going to Sri Lanka. I would book the plane tickets the following week.

We were worried about how our families would react when they heard we were planning to elope. The expectation would be for a proper Irish wedding. If we didn't book the plane tickets, we'd be persuaded to stay, I was sure of it. We needed to get those tickets.

We finalised our travel dates and made out an itinerary. As I picked up my diary to put the dates into the calendar, a thought suddenly struck me. I counted out the days of the month since my last period. I was late. It couldn't be, I thought. I had just stopped taking the pill a few weeks beforehand.

I got into the car and went to the chemist to buy a pregnancy test. When I got home I went straight upstairs to take it. I watched as the window filled up. One pink line emerged, and then ... two. Three minutes later I came down the stairs, crying.

'What's wrong, Vicky?' Jim looked surprised.

I took a breath. 'I'm pregnant,' I said, holding up the test.

I'll never forget the look on his face at that moment: pure happiness. He was going to be a dad.

'What do we do now?' I asked. We laughed. Neither of us knew. It's funny, you can know a lot of people who've had babies, but it's all a bit of a mystery until you're going through it yourself. What did people do after they found out they were pregnant? I read somewhere that you should go to your GP, so I went to the GP to have a check-up and to tell her I was pregnant, to get her advice. She took my blood pressure and gave me a leaflet with all the dos and don'ts. Then she asked me a few questions.

'Do you smoke?'

'No.'

'Do you drink alcohol?'

'Not now that I'm pregnant.'

'Are you thinking of travelling anytime soon?'

'Yes'

'Ah ...'

That was the clincher. I started to tell her all about Sri Lanka, about the plans for the wedding, the great adventure, the beaches and the jungle and the blue train that snakes through the countryside. Then I stopped. She was looking at me in a way that said there was something she didn't want to have to tell me.

'What is it?' I asked.

'Well … you would need vaccinations for Sri Lanka and I'm afraid …'

My face fell.

'… you won't be able to have any vaccinations while you're pregnant.'

I paused for a moment. 'I suppose scuba diving is out of the question then?' I asked.

She laughed. 'I'm afraid so.'

I couldn't believe this was all happening. I had heard it would probably take time to become pregnant, up to six months, after coming off the pill. Ever the planner, I had decided to stop taking the pill in October, thinking that by the time we were married in March, we'd be ready for a baby. It was only December, and I was pregnant already, a few months ahead of schedule. It wasn't exactly how we planned it, but then again, most things aren't.

We needed to rethink the whole elopement idea. That night Jim and I talked it all through and came up with a plan. We tried to imagine a place that would be like Sri Lanka but wouldn't require vaccinations. So I did what I do best, I began researching. That's where the idea of St Lucia came from. It was a small volcanic island in the Caribbean with mountains and beautiful sandy beaches that stretch as far as the eye can see. It was settled. We would get married in St Lucia.

15

Wedding Bells

S T LUCIA WAS EVERYTHING WE dreamed it would be: an island paradise. It was like being transported to a world of technicolour – the palm trees were blowing in the wind, the Afro-Caribbean music blared from the car radios and we marvelled at the colourful clothing of people along the streets selling coconuts and manning busy market stalls. I loved the feel of the cool ocean breeze against my skin as it pushed through the warm midday air. We gave ourselves a few days to explore the island before the big day.

Then finally the day arrived – 9 March 2005. That morning I woke up feeling excited. Jim went to the hotel to give me some space while I got dressed in our apartment. The day was hot. I laid my wedding dress out carefully on the bed, took a deep breath, then put it on, hoping it would fit. I was now ten weeks pregnant. Mam and I had shopped for the dress and we found a beautiful simple coral two-piece in Monsoon. I zipped it up, slowly. It fit perfectly.

I looked at my reflection in the mirror. This was it: my wedding day. My only regret was that I wished Mam and Lyndsey were with me. I always imagined I would be with them getting ready on the morning of my wedding. The rest of the bells and whistles of the day mattered very little to me. But I knew they would have made getting ready very special. I imagined Lyndsey styling my hair and making me feel loved and looked after, the way she always does. And Mam would have fussed over me, and made us both laugh.

But they weren't there. This is what we had decided to do. I needed to make my peace with that and make it a happy day for both of us. After all, we were in paradise. And we only had each other to make it special.

I needed to be at the beach for twelve o'clock. I put on my gold sandals and walked out under the palm trees, feeling the heat of the sun on my skin. I followed the path to the beach. It was a beautiful day. The waves were gently lapping onto the shore. I reached the clearing and when I turned the corner, there was Jim. He was near the water, standing under an arch made out of white satin cloth and wood from the surrounding trees. I walked towards him slowly, smiling. I saw his eyes fill up with tears. I reached the makeshift altar and took his hands in mine.

'You look beautiful,' he said.

The celebrant was a large Caribbean man with a great big smile and a booming voice. He had the kind of smile that made you smile. He talked about what marriage meant and why it was such an important thing to do. We said our vows, our promises to one another – for richer, for poorer, in sickness and in health. And then he pronounced us man and wife. We kissed, feeling the warm sand under our feet and listening to the ocean rejoicing behind us. And just like that, we were married.

We had a special candlelit dinner that evening, looking out over the bay. The waiters brought champagne to the table. Jim was drinking it for two. But we were both sun-kissed and drunk on life.

We spent two blissful weeks in St Lucia and a week in Barbados before returning home for the celebrations. When we came back we organised a family gathering, a homecoming to mark the occasion. We held a big party in Jim's parents' pub surrounded by family and friends. We raised a glass to toast our life together, may it be happy and full of love, in the company of family and friends. The champagne flowed and we danced late into the night.

The start of our journey as husband and wife.

16

Amelia

OVER THE MONTHS THAT FOLLOWED, I watched my bump grow. I loved feeling the little kicks inside my stomach, knowing my little one was going to be feisty and determined, just like their mam. It was such a strange concept to think that a person was growing inside of me – a little piece of me and a little piece of Jim. I couldn't wait to meet our baby. I tried to stay healthy, to do all the right things.

As the months went by we began to prepare for the new arrival. Mam was knitting cardigans – white and lemon – as we didn't know yet if it would be a boy or girl, and we were busy choosing baby things: a buggy and clothes, such as tiny socks and Baby-gros.

When I was twenty-eight weeks pregnant it was time for a routine check-up with my gynaecologist. We had chosen to get private healthcare given my medical history. I had shattered my pelvis in the accident and had been told that I would probably have difficult pregnancies.

Everything had been going really well. I was checking in with the gynaecologist regularly and I had managed to stay active for the first six months of the pregnancy. I was swimming again and was feeling healthy and fit as I drove into Waterford for the appointment. My hair was still damp as I had come straight from the pool.

I lay back in the chair. The consultant placed the cold jelly on my stomach and rolled the ultrasound instrument over my skin. I looked up at the screen as he moved back and forth across my stomach. I looked at his expression. He seemed concerned, adjusting the ultrasound and looking intently at the screen.

'What is it?' I asked. I knew something was wrong. In my last scan, you could clearly make out the baby's head and body and little feet and toes. Now, on the screen the baby looked less clear, full of black circles.

'I'm just going to have another look here,' he said, presumably not wanting to alarm me.

We were both silent for the next few minutes as he rolled the gel across my stomach and activated the scan again. 'Is your husband coming in today?' he asked, tentatively.

'No,' I replied.

'Is he nearby?'

'He's working,' I said, becoming nervous by the line of questioning.

'It might be a good idea to give him a call ...'

'Is everything okay?'

'I am going to have to admit you, I'm afraid. We need to run some tests. I don't like what I am seeing on the scan. There is a lot of fluid around your baby's abdomen. Once you have been admitted, I will call down to you this evening when I know more.'

I stepped outside and made the call. My hands were shaking. 'Jim, you need to get in here.'

'Vicky, are you alright? Is it the baby?'

'There's something wrong with the baby. I'm being admitted.'

Jim was standing on a roof working on a building job when I called. He hung up, climbed down the scaffolding and got straight into the car without saying a word to anyone. I was sitting in admissions when he came through the door. His face had aged, if that was possible, since I had seen him that morning at breakfast.

They admitted me to the gynaecological ward. I hadn't been in hospital since the accident. It was bringing back memories of that time – the sense of powerlessness, of desperation. There was a deep sadness I kept locked away, a box I never dared to open – the pain and loss of Christophe and the trauma of the accident. Being in hospital was the closest I had come to opening up those emotions again. I was put in a semi-private room but the other bed was empty. I was thankful for this as I wasn't in the humour for talking to anyone.

The nurses came to take my bloods and they placed a baby monitor on my stomach to track the baby's activity. I could hear my baby's heartbeat, strong and steady. The noise was comforting.

'There's no easy way to say this,' the doctor said, coming into the room later that evening. 'I know you must be worried so I'll get to the point quickly. I'm afraid I am seeing some significant abnormalities on your scan.'

'What do you mean, abnormalities?' I asked.

'This isn't going to be a straightforward birth.'

'What is it?' I asked.

He told us that it was likely that our baby would either have a congenital heart defect, Edwards' syndrome or toxoplasmosis, all very serious disorders. 'It's hard to know yet … we will have to wait for the results of the blood tests to come back. In the meantime, I really can't let you go home until we know what we are dealing with so we will keep you here and monitor your baby's activity.'

The results came back two weeks later. It was toxoplasmosis, a disease caused by a parasite called the toxoplasma gondii. In pregnancy, the danger of contracting toxoplasmosis is that if the infection is passed on to the baby in the womb, the baby's immune system cannot fight off the parasite and so the parasite attacks the eyes and the brain. The worst-case scenario was that my baby would be born blind and severely brain-damaged.

The doctor told us that he had never dealt with toxoplasmosis before but that he was consulting with specialists in Wales and he would make sure he was up to date on the best ways to treat it.

While I was in hospital, we decided to find out the sex of the baby. I needed something to keep me going so we asked the consultant to tell us at one of my scans. 'It's a girl,' he said, smiling.

'A little girl!' I said, rubbing my stomach. 'Hello, little one, we can't wait to meet you.' I clung to this bit of news, as I was finding being in hospital very unnerving. I wasn't sleeping and was worried all the time. At least now I could try to imagine my little girl.

The days on the ward were long. Across the hall was another patient, who always stopped to say hello. She came into my room as she was passing and asked me how my appointment had gone.

Me at 6 months old with Mam
at Nanny Kelly's house,
April 1975.

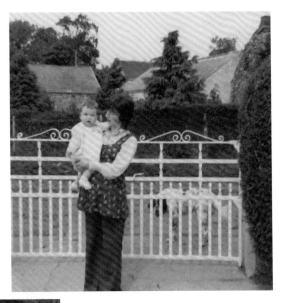

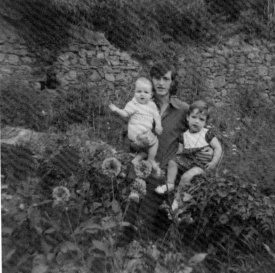

Me (right) at age two-and
a-half, with Dad and my
brother Robbie, at home
in Ballygorey, summer
1977.

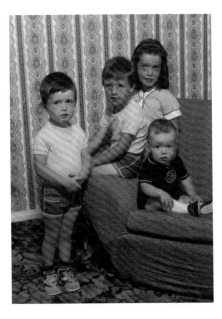

Me with my brothers Lee
(standing), Robbie and baby
Jonnie in our living room
in Mooncoin, 1981.

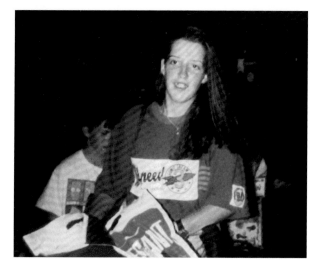

Returning home from France after my first summer spent working as an au pair aged 16, August 1991.

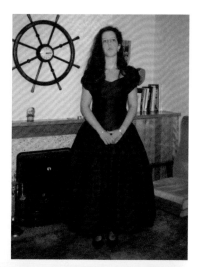

The glamour of a 1990s' Debs!

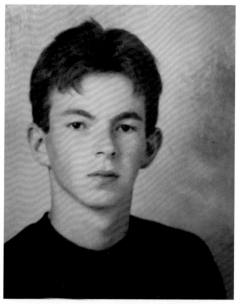

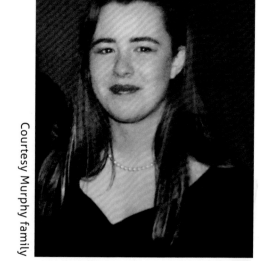

Christophe, my boyfriend, and Lisa, a friend, were tragically killed in a car accident which I was very lucky to survive, July 1994.

Recovering from my accident in France: in my geriatric wheelchair at Waterford Regional Hospital August/September 1994.

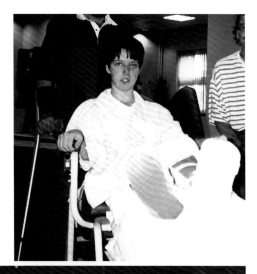

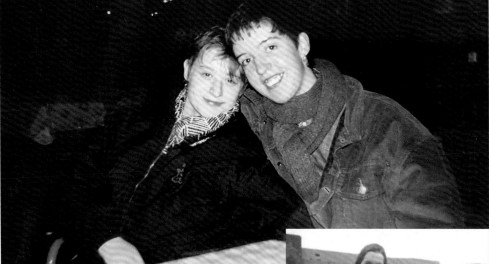

Me and Katy pictured one year after the car accident at a rehabilitation centre in Berck-sur-Mer, France, 1995.

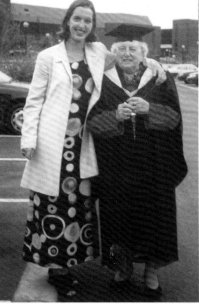

Sharing a proud moment with Nanny Fitzgerald (who enjoyed donning my cap and gown!) – graduating with a BA in European Studies at University of Limerick in 1997.

With my future husband Jim – our last night together before he left for his trip to Australia, August 1997.

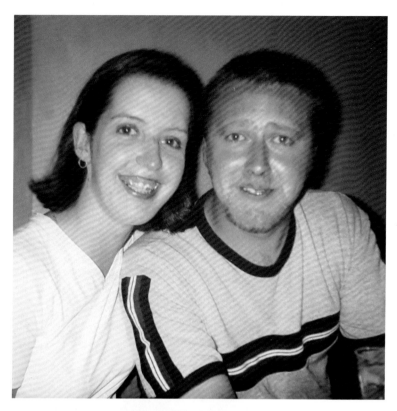

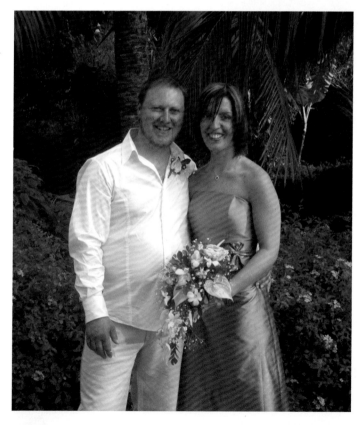

Our 'getaway wedding' – St Lucia, 9 March 2005.

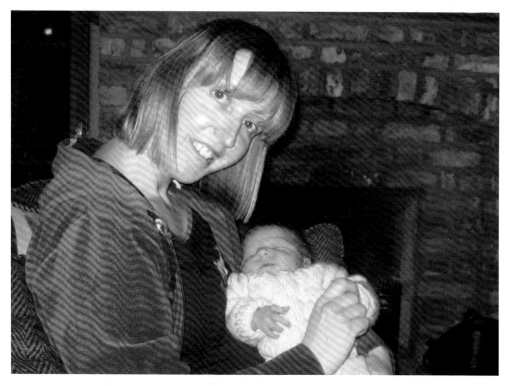

The start of a new journey with the arrival of our beautiful baby Amelia, 2005.

And, five-and-a-half years on, another precious arrival – our son, Darragh.

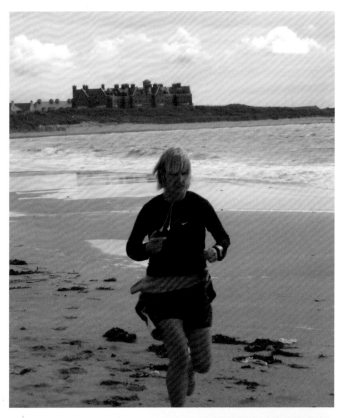

Combining my two favourite pleasures – running and the beach at Doughmore – as I train for my first marathon in June 2007.

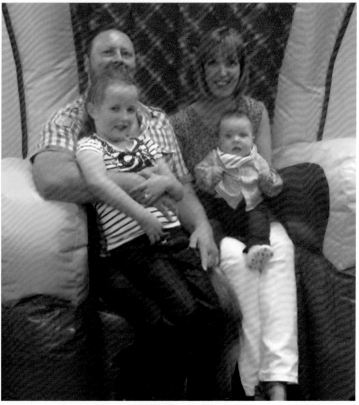

Celebrating Amelia's 6th birthday, August 2011. A couple of months earlier, I had had the smear test that changed everything. I had been told it was clear but, when audited, the result was changed to squamous cell carcinoma. I had cancer in this photo and it would be three years' later before I knew it.

Amelia's First Holy Communion in April 2014 – less than two months before I discovered I had cancer for the first time.

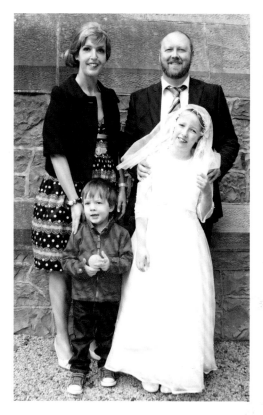

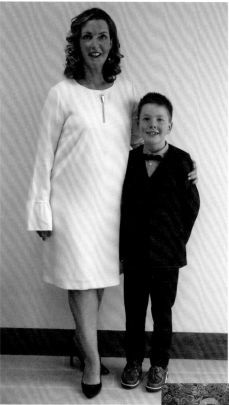

Darragh and I on his Communion day in April 2019.

Me with my sister Lyndsey, our kids, her partner Matty, and Mam and Dad, visiting Santa at Birr Castle in December 2017. I knew my cancer had returned but decided to wait to tell my family until after Christmas.

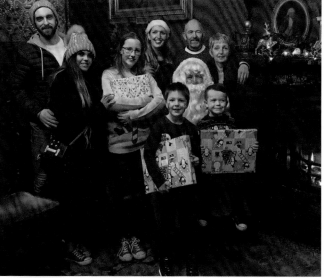

Darragh's 'Free Writing Exercise' for his teacher about his mammy's cancer, May 2018. It says: 'My mommy has cancer and she won't die cus she is taking drugs and her juice. So that what happened. And then she was ok. And I keep care of her and today she is going to Galway and then Dublin. And in a few months she might be going to America.'

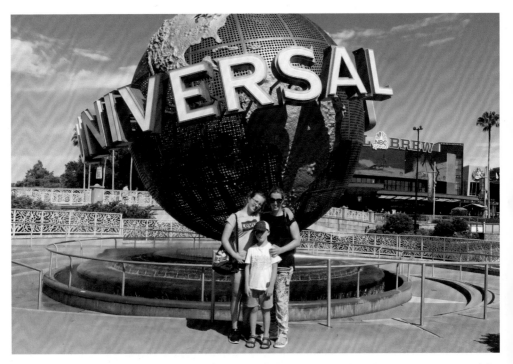

Myself and the kids at Universal Studios, Orlando, on a memorable family trip, August 2018.

'They've diagnosed me with something and they're worried about the baby,' I said.

'What did they say it was?' she asked.

'It's something not many people have heard of,' I explained, not wanting to get drawn on the detail.

'Toxoplasmosis?'

'Yes,' I said. 'How did you know?'

'I had that,' she said, 'when I was seven. I woke up one day and I couldn't see with my left eye.'

I looked at her, studied her properly for the first time since I'd been on the ward, trying to take her in.

'I turned out okay, though, didn't I?' she said, smiling. 'It will be okay. She'll be just fine,' she added, reassuringly.

I felt like she had been sent from above. Like a guardian angel.

'What's your name?' I asked.

'Amelia,' she smiled. And with that, she was gone.

During my three-week stint in Waterford Regional, the consultant sent me to Holles Street in Dublin for an amniocentesis. Jim drove me to the appointment. There wasn't much conversation; we were both lost in thought. When we got to the hospital, I lay back in the chair for the procedure and pulled up my top. I hated the thought of the long needle piercing my body, but tried to concentrate on what it was for. This would give our baby the best chance. It was something that had to be done. We needed to be sure of the diagnosis before I started taking medication for it.

Two doctors came into the room, a neonatologist who deals specifically with high-risk pregnancies, and his assistant, a female doctor. 'Hello, Mrs Phelan. Are you all set? Have my team explained the procedure to you?' he asked.

'Yes,' I said. I wondered why the consultants are so often men, at the point where you feel most vulnerable as a woman.

He took the needle out of the box and started the ultrasound. My baby appeared on the screen in front of me. She was there with us in the room – a reminder that she was on the way. It was all going to be alright. I had to keep telling myself that.

'Hmmm ...'

'What was that?' I asked.

'... just, if you lived in the UK, you could consider having a termination.'

I felt numb. The needle pierced through my skin.

'Okay, deep breath,' he said.

I could feel the tears rolling down my cheeks. Jim was squeezing my hand. I closed my eyes tight, wishing for it to be over.

'What are you suggesting?' I asked, shaking. 'Are you telling me that my baby is not going to survive?'

'There is no way of knowing for sure. I was merely saying that some patients consider going to the UK for terminations. The results will be sent to your gynaecologist.'

With that, he removed his gloves with a snap and left the room. I didn't move. I stayed lying on the chair, my face red and tear-stained. I could feel the eyes of the female doctor on me. I didn't look at her. I couldn't. I just wanted to get out of there.

I gathered myself together and left the room. I was crying now. I could hardly catch my breath. Jim was holding me close to his chest. The other women in the waiting room were watching me with concerned looks on their faces. The female doctor followed us out.

'Mrs Phelan, wait,' she said. 'Please come with me. There is a family room down the corridor where you can have some privacy.' She led us to a room with a sofa, and a crucifix on the wall. I was inconsolable at this stage. Once I managed to stop crying, I felt angry.

'Who does he think he is?' I said. 'How dare he! I am thirty weeks pregnant.' I pointed at my swollen belly. 'Look at me! Why would I come all the way up here to have an amniocentesis if I didn't want to have this baby?'

'I understand. I'm very sorry, Mrs Phelan.'

With that, the neonatologist entered the room. He had obviously been told that I was upset. 'Mrs Phelan, you seem very distressed.'

'Of course I'm distressed. Are you trying to tell me that this baby is not going to be compatible with life?' I was speaking loudly now. He looked uncomfortable, probably wondering if the patients in the waiting room could hear the conversation. I raised my voice again. 'Why do you think I would drive all the way from Waterford and put myself through that amniocentesis if I didn't want this baby?'

'Mrs Phelan ...'

'Get out!' I screamed.

I felt so angry. All I had hoped for was a healthy baby. I had done everything I could to bring her safely into the world. And I wasn't going to stop now. How dare he suggest that I terminate my pregnancy. He knew nothing about me. And anyway, he couldn't be one hundred per cent sure that this baby was not going to be okay.

My gynaecologist put me on a lot of medication once the results came back. It was confirmed: our baby had toxoplasmosis. She was the first baby in Ireland ever to be diagnosed with toxoplasmosis in the womb.

'It'll be a learning curve,' he said. 'But we'll do everything we can.' He was very reassuring and I trusted him with my baby's life .

I got home from the chemist and placed all the boxes of tablets on the table. The kitchen looked like a pharmacy. I would have to take forty-five tablets a day. The side-effects were very difficult; they were making me vomit. The only thing that seemed to steady my stomach was lying down. I stayed in bed for long periods of time; some days I barely got up at all. I lay there looking at the ceiling. I was starting to feel depressed. I was full of fear for what might happen to the baby.

Just when I thought things couldn't get any worse I started to develop a rash on my chest and on the palms of my hands. Mam was in the kitchen. She had her glasses on and was examining the back of the pill packets when I came down the stairs. 'Show me your hands again,' she said. I showed her my hands. They were raw red with a rash that ran up my arms and across my chest.

'It's getting worse,' I said, as I made for the loo again to be sick.

I called my gynaecologist's office to make an appointment. I explained to his secretary, Mary, that I had developed a rash. She called me back within an hour to tell me to come in the following morning.

Mam came with me. We sat in front of the doctor and showed him the rash and asked him if it was a side-effect from the medication.

'Vicky, I don't know how to tell you this except to say that there's a strong possibility that you have obstetric cholestasis. I mean, we will have to get bloods done today to confirm but looking at the rash you have and the fact that you are vomiting bile, I am pretty sure that's what you have.'

This meant that suddenly there was a much higher chance of me miscarrying. If the bile leaked into the amniotic fluid, it could kill the baby. I didn't know what to say.

My mother was inconsolable. She feared the worst.

The doctor explained that he was going to bring me in at thirty-seven weeks to induce me. I was now thirty-six weeks pregnant.

I felt partly relieved by the fact that they would induce me. I was ready for this nightmare pregnancy to be over. I needed to meet my baby so that I knew she was safely delivered and we could take care of her.

I was admitted to hospital a few days later, where they induced me. I started pacing the corridor in my dressing gown. 'Walk, Vicky,' a friend had told me. 'Keep walking.' So that's what I did.

Five hours later, I was in labour. I was pushing for just under an hour. And then she arrived, at 5.50 p.m. A beautiful little bundle, weighing just 5 pounds 12 ounces. We named her Amelia.

I had never loved anyone as much as I loved her, instantly. I held her in my arms as I breastfed her. I looked at her, wondering if she would open her eyes and be able to look back at me. We knew that toxoplasmosis could cause blindness. It would be a few months before they would know whether or not she was able to see.

I held her tight and kissed her forehead. 'You're going to be okay, Amelia. Mammy's here. It's going to be okay.' I cradled her in my arms, and wondered what her life would be like. Who she would turn out to be.

My baby. My little Amelia.

17

And Then There Were Three

THEY TELL YOU THAT it's a big life change, but you're never really prepared for how big it is and how all-encompassing it is: parenthood. Motherhood, to be exact.

The day we brought Amelia home from the hospital was the start of a new life for all of us. We were a family now. Life had meaning in a way it never had before. The house even felt different. It felt less like a house, and more like a home. Her home.

I brought her up to my bedroom and lay with her in my arms and closed my eyes for a moment. I thought of the doctor who had spoken of terminating the pregnancy. I would like to see him now and show him my beautiful little girl. I thought of that angel, Amelia, in the hospital ward who told us everything would be okay. I thought of the midwives who had helped to deliver her safely. She didn't know it yet, but all these people had played a part in her journey into the world. And here she was: our world.

It all started out well. We were doing our best, learning how to cope with a newborn baby, but as the weeks and months wore on, things started to take a turn. Mam came over to help when she could. We were getting by. Like any young couple with a baby we were surviving on very little sleep, but Amelia's condition made caring for her more complicated.

She cried a lot, sometimes all through the night. She was very colicky and was on a lot of medication. We had to accept that she probably couldn't see very much. She was floppy too as her muscles hadn't developed in the way that they should have, which made her neck very delicate. We had to be extra careful with her. We tried to do everything right.

It was getting exhausting. No matter what we did, she cried. It frustrated me when she wouldn't settle or sleep. I was losing patience. I felt myself starting to go down. I was snapping at Jim. I hadn't slept in months.

I was going back and forth to Mam's every day, or she was coming over to my house to help with the baby. I was bringing Amelia to the hospital three days a week to have injections. Getting into the car upset Amelia, so I learned how to inject one of her medicines, Neupogen, so that we didn't have to go to the hospital so much. She needed this injection three times a week.

I felt like I was sleepwalking, moving mindlessly from one day to the next. I didn't care about anything anymore. I couldn't see a way out of the constant exhaustion and misery. Every day was consumed with crying and nappies and medication.

People tried to give me advice. Other mums would talk to me about the best ways to put a baby to sleep, or how to get the baby to stop crying, but their advice frustrated me. They made it sound so easy, but they didn't understand. None of them had a baby with a congenital condition. This was different. She wasn't an ordinary baby.

I had lost a lot of weight. I didn't feel like eating anymore. I forgot to eat most of the time, until Mam or Jim reminded me. Then I would have a slice of toast or something small, just for the sake of it. I didn't find pleasure in it anymore.

One day Jim came in from work, and threw his keys down on the hall table, as he always did. Amelia was crying again. The incessant screams and wails could be heard throughout the house. I was still breastfeeding at the time. Sometimes I felt she could sense I wasn't happy, that she could feel my depression, and it made her cry even more. No matter how hard I tried, I couldn't get her to settle.

Jim came into the room. 'How is she?' he asked. With that, I started to cry. I handed her to him. 'I've had enough!' I said, taking the car keys from the hall table.

I could see the look of panic on Jim's face. 'Where are you going?' he said.

'I don't know. Anywhere. I just need to get away or I will fucking kill her. I will actually kill her.' I got into the car, reversed dangerously fast out of the driveway, and went speeding down the hill. I drove for miles. I stopped eventually at the river and pulled over. I collapsed onto the steering wheel and fell apart. It was all too much.

Jim must have told Mam about the incident. She was at the house the following morning, and I could sense she was watching me, cautiously gauging my behaviour. 'You'll have to stop breastfeeding,' she said, as I lifted Amelia off my chest after her feed, carefully cradling her neck to support her. 'You're going to kill yourself if you keep going on like this.' I stopped breastfeeding that week. I had lost so much weight that my body felt weak and needed to recover. I also needed some time away.

The University of Limerick had emailed me a few weeks beforehand with an offer of some consultancy work in their International Office, an email I hadn't responded to. I got in touch with them and told them I was available to work immediately. I packed my bags and went to Limerick the following week to work from their offices for a few days. I was running away again. I knew it, but I needed to do it. I had to get out of that house before I went mad.

Mam minded Amelia while I was gone. I was in Limerick for five days and though it is hard to admit, I didn't miss her, even for a moment. I could breathe for the first time in a long time. I stayed in an apartment on campus and caught up with old friends. I was back at work, and I loved it. Sitting in the office checking off my task list was invigorating. I was surrounded by adult company again. I was presenting in meetings and meeting deadlines, filing reports and using my brain once more.

The week went all too quickly and before I knew it, it was time to go back home to Kilkenny to pick up Amelia. 'Come in for a cup of tea,' Mam said, welcoming me at the door. 'She's missed you!' She gestured towards Amelia, who was lying in her cot. I looked in at her briefly and went to make a cup of tea.

'How was she?' I asked.

Mam started filling me in on how many hours sleep she'd had each night and how her medication dispensing had gone. We were very quickly back to baby talk. Amelia started crying softly, which soon turned into a wail. I put my head in my hands. Back to reality.

'The child is crying,' Mam said, waiting for me to react. I didn't move. Mam got up to pick Amelia up. She cradled her close to her chest and bounced her in her arms. 'Shhhhh, it's okay, Amelia … shhhhh.'

'I better go,' I said, putting the cups in the sink.

Dad helped me to gather all of Amelia's things and put them in the car. He fastened the baby seat and Mam carried Amelia out, swaddled in the knitted blanket she had made for her. She handed her to me. Then I realised there were tears in her eyes – Mam's, not the baby's. She could see how I looked at Amelia. It was breaking her heart to hand her back to me, knowing I was not in a position to love her the way I should.

As I drove away, I looked at Amelia through the rear-view mirror, lying in the baby seat in the back of the car. I tried to work out what I was feeling towards her. It was resentment; I resented her for bringing this depression into my life.

None of it made sense. She was everything I could ever have hoped for. I loved her unconditionally. But no matter how hard I tried, I couldn't bring myself to feel joy with her. Eventually I had to face up to the facts. I had post-natal depression. Even the idea of it was foreign to me. I couldn't understand why I would be depressed after having a baby.

I went to see the doctor. It wasn't my usual GP. As I sat across from him I realised how difficult it would be to explain what I was going through. How could someone not judge a mum who couldn't love her newborn baby?

'How can I help you today?' he said.

I cleared my throat. He looked at me, waiting for a reply. I had to say something, anything.

'I've been feeling very down lately …' I said eventually.

The doctor shuffled in his chair. 'Okay, and have you experienced any major life events recently? Anything that might have caused this reaction?'

'I had a baby four months ago and I've been feeling this way ever since.'

He placed me on the weighing scales and took a blood sample. 'Have you been eating regularly?' he asked.

'No,' I said.

He scribbled something on his notepad, tore off the docket and handed me a script. 'I'm going to start you on these and see how you get on,' he said.

I looked at the piece of paper. Anti-depressants. I waited for further instructions. None came. I was hoping he was going to adopt some kind of holistic approach – that I could combine medication with lifestyle changes. There was no talk of meditation or exercise. Just a box of pills to meddle with the chemicals of my malfunctioning brain.

For several days the box of anti-depressants sat on my bedside table, unopened. I was reluctant to take them as I was afraid of how they might change me.

After one particularly long day with Amelia, when I was feeling really worn out, I poured a glass of water and took two of the tablets before going to bed. Anything had to be better than this, I told myself.

I took them for two weeks but felt myself going down further. They didn't seem to be working for me, so I stopped them, cold turkey. I never heard from the doctor. No one rang to see how I was getting on or to tell me to come in for a six-week check-up or anything. But, I suppose, why would they? I was in this alone. It was up to me to find the answer. No one could make me happy but me.

I needed to make some changes in my life. A job came up in Waterford Institute of Technology in the adult literacy department, which I decided to apply for. I got the job. Amelia was now six months old and Mam had offered to mind her for me if I decided to go back to work. I was so grateful to my mother for giving me this lifeline. I felt that getting back to work would help me to feel myself again, and it did. Being in the working world helped to give me a new focus, a new sense of self.

One of my new colleagues had suggested I give acupuncture a go. She said it worked wonders for her when she was getting over the fatigue of pregnancy. I hadn't told her I was depressed, but I wondered if she sensed it. It was still a secret I tried to keep hidden from the rest of the world. I couldn't understand it, so how could I expect others to? It was like I was leading a double life – trying to put my best self forward in work, and then when I came home at night, my demons caught up with me. I was hard to be around. It wasn't easy for Jim, with all the responsibilities that parenthood brings, to have to deal with my depression as well.

A few days later I found myself lying on a massage table with needles sticking into me. The man administrating the acupuncture talked in hushed, reassuring tones as the needles pierced through my skin, one by one. The acupuncture helped. I had more energy after it. Though, lying down for an hour may have had something to do with it too!

I started reading up about post-natal depression. I wanted to understand what was happening to my body and mind and what I could do to reverse it. I needed to do it, for myself and for Amelia. We were a team in life, and she needed me to be fully present, to be the best mother I could be. I owed that to her. And to myself.

I tried everything. I bought myself one of those light boxes, that simulates the light of the sun. I set it up in the sitting room.

'What on earth are you doing?' asked Jim, walking in to find me sitting in the armchair under a cold blue light.

'I'm boosting my serotonin,' I said casually. He didn't ask any more questions. I sat under the light all through the winter, using it on my desk in the office at work. At home I put it on in the mornings and evenings. It came with instructions for the recommended time to use it. The light it emits is the blue light we are lacking in the northern hemisphere. I was sceptical at first, but reckoned it couldn't do any harm.

I read everything I could get my hands on about post-natal depression. It's how I deal with anything – read as much as I can about it. I found an online forum on an English website. It was a forum for mums who were suffering from the condition. I would spend hours reading the posts, being a voyeur, learning about other people's experiences. It made me feel less alone. One day I invented an alias. I wrote my first post about my own experience.

As it was the internet, I could be completely anonymous. It meant I could be as honest as I liked. I couldn't explain what I was going through to anyone in my 'real' life, I was too ashamed. But online I was able to speak openly for the first time, about how I was feeling and what I was doing to combat it. I pressed 'send' and waited nervously for a reply.

The next morning I logged in again and scrolled down the page, as I always did. There it was: my post – in black and white for the world to see. And underneath it were several replies. Other mums had written to empathise with my situation. They had gone through many of the same experiences. Some were out the other side, others were still going through it. I breathed a sigh of relief. It made a huge difference to be able to verbalise what I was feeling, to know it was normal, in a way, and that other people had felt the same way I did, and had come through it.

People didn't necessarily have the answers. They might just be able to tell you that it's okay to feel that way, or give you some advice based on their experiences. It made me feel less alone and gave me the hope I needed to get myself back on track. It made all the difference when someone gave me a bit of hope. It helped me get through the day.

It was around that time that I took up running. One of the mums on the forum talked about how much it had helped her through her post-natal depression. I bought a good pair of trainers and went for my first outing. I came back feeling full of energy. I started going every day. Jim minded Amelia while I went. He could see it was helping to boost my mood, so he encouraged me to get out the door in the mornings.

I came home one morning after my run with a great idea. I needed a challenge, something to train for. At first I considered signing up to a 10k run, but no, it needed to be something bigger. I was going to run a marathon. I mapped out a training plan, with daily and weekly goals. It was like the Leaving Cert all over again. I was on a mission. I never missed a day – I'd run in the morning, I'd run during my lunch break, I'd run home, or back to my mother's. I worked my life around running.

Running was my saviour, my saving grace for a long time. I think it was a combination of the time on my own, and the exercise creating endorphins. I felt healthy and good in my body and I had never been as fit. I was just a nicer person to be around. If I had any stress, I ran it out of me. No matter where I was, no matter how I was feeling, I brought my runners and my running gear and ran until I felt better.

I even joined a running group in Waterford near work. It

gave me a good social outlet, with other people who loved running. On my first day with them they were getting ready to run thirteen miles. It was my first time doing that kind of distance and I was a bit nervous I wouldn't be able to keep up. A couple of the older men hung back to encourage me along.

'Come on now, Vicky, you can do it,' they said.

And I did. I crossed the finish line. The others all high-fived me as I ran the last few feet. It felt incredible to be part of something again.

I was never one for team sports, but I loved the positive energy and camaraderie. A little time to escape and run.

From then on, we went on thirteen-mile runs every Saturday and I completed my first marathon in Belfast in May 2008 in a time of 4.00.08. Those extra eight seconds nearly killed me as I had been hoping for a sub-four-hour marathon, but the feeling I got crossing the finish line was like nothing I had ever experienced before.

The running helped a great deal and though I was starting to feel a little better, it took nearly a year before the fog of depression lifted and I felt like my old self again.

The happier I was in my own skin, the better mother I could be for Amelia. I needed to do that for her, to be the mother she deserved. I made a promise to myself that I would never let Amelia down, no matter how I was feeling. And somehow, even on the darkest days, I managed to keep that promise. I brought her to every appointment in the hospital – often three or four times a week for various therapies – and always made sure she had everything she needed. I never felt fully present through it – I was going through the motions – but I was there, I showed up for her, I made sure of that. And now I was even starting to enjoy life again. I felt lighter in myself; the darkness was starting to pass and she was happier because of it. Babies are very instinctive. I think she could sense my pain and it was making her upset. Now we were both happier in ourselves. And she was making great progress.

We also found out that she was able to see, though her sight would always be compromised. She was partially blind in her right eye and we would have to monitor the situation closely, as there was still a danger she could go blind one day. It was a huge relief to both of us to know that she had some vision. I swore to myself that, no matter what it took, we needed to make sure she was always able to see, to save her from a life of blindness. If it took everything in me, I would be there to make sure of that.

One day as I was walking through town, on a break from work, I went to the book shop. I thumbed through the titles on the shelves and found what I was looking for, a book called *The Road Less Travelled*. A woman on the forum had recommended it. One of the opening lines is:

Life is difficult. This is a great truth, one of the greatest truths. It is a great truth because once we truly see this truth, we transcend it.

The moment I read those words, something inside me clicked. Sometimes I looked at all the things that had happened in my life and wondered: why are things always happening to me? Why is my life so difficult? The big premise of that book is that life in general is unfair – just accept it and get over it and move on. You'll have to deal with it, because that's a part of life. It helped me to see things in a new way. Sometimes I felt like I had been given a bad roll of the dice – that life had been particularly unfair to me, between the accident and Amelia's condition. But life was like that for everyone, in one way or another. Everyone knows pain during their lifetime, and it is a part of the acceptance of what life is about. I felt lighter after reading those lines, as if I wasn't battling a lone war. Everyone was on the front line, and we needed to help each other, it's what makes us human. We were in it together.

The book helped me to realise that I needed to go to counselling. Though I knew it would be a big part of helping to keep my depression at bay, I didn't have the courage at that time to go and talk to someone. It was nearly a year later, in 2007, when I finally decided to talk to someone professionally. Waterford Institute of Technology offered staff members eight free sessions of counselling, which allowed me the opportunity to go and talk about everything I had been through.

Sometimes all the counsellor is doing is listening to you. But sometimes that's all you need, someone to listen. It wasn't easy, though, especially at first. My initial sessions were challenging. In the very first session I opened up to the counsellor about the car accident. After that, she seemed to fixate on it. 'Do you think those feelings go back to the time of your car accident?' she would ask.

I felt like no matter what we were talking about, she brought it back to the accident. One day I'd had enough. We were talking about my depression after Amelia's birth. 'What does this have to do with my accident?' I barked.

'Everything, Vicky,' she said.

Over time I realised she was right. I was still harbouring a lot of pain from that time in my life – from the close brush with death and the loss of my friends. In theory I had moved on, grown up, got married and had a child. To the onlooker I seemed to be doing well, excelling in college and in my field of work, but underneath it, the scars ran deep. And these things have a way of catching up with you. The emotions were still there and were manifesting themselves in different ways, in the way I was dealing with motherhood, in the way I was relating to my husband. This realisation helped me to turn a corner. Knowing why something is happening goes a long way to understanding how to stop it.

Counselling can be frightening, peeling back the layers, like peeling an onion, while your eyes stream with tears. But it's worth the sting, when you get to the heart of things. It's only then that you begin to heal.

18

A New Chapter Of Life

AS TIME PASSED WE STARTED to feel more settled. Three years had gone by and I was really enjoying my job in the literacy department. I worked with a wonderful team of supportive women who I was able to be open and honest with and who helped me through some of my darkest days. For the first time in my life, I felt a part of something that really mattered. We were responsible for designing, developing and delivering programmes for those working with people with low literacy levels – people who had had a bad experience of the education system, others who couldn't read or write at all and wanted to learn, or some who just wanted to be able to help their kids with their homework. Education had been my lifeline. I knew what a difference it could make to people's lives.

I felt very lucky to have my mother to mind Amelia while I worked. It gave me peace of mind to know she was being looked after. With all her hospital appointments and medication, I would not have been able to go back to work without Mam's help. Nobody else would have taken on a child like Amelia.

Every evening, I would pick Amelia up from my parents' house on my way home. She was always running around, playing with toys and, as soon as she was old enough, Mam was encouraging her to read. It reminded me of being at home when I was a child. It was a happy house. Mam was always knitting something new for Amelia – a scarf or a hat – and Dad would have made some sort of new contraption for her to play with. She loved being there and I could see she was really coming out of herself.

I wasn't sure I could have got through those years without Mam and Dad close by, being there, helping me through. But we had made it, and we were in a good place as a family. I was feeling much better, but I was keeping an eye on things, being careful to look for signs that my mood might be changing.

Mam and I watched Amelia playing one Sunday afternoon while we had a cup of tea at the kitchen table.

'Would you not think about having another one?' Mam asked me. I could tell she had been thinking a lot about it.

'Ah, I don't know …' I said, stirring my tea.

Mam had seen how difficult the first pregnancy was. 'I'd love for you to know what pregnancy is like without the complications,' she continued.

'I know,' I said. 'I just worry.' The thoughts of being so sick again and of the baby being sick again were almost too much for me.

'But do you want Amelia to be an only child?' she asked.

I looked at Amelia playing on her own. I definitely didn't want that.

'And we'd be here to help,' she said. And I knew they would. They always were.

A few months later, in the summer of 2010, I was pregnant. The timing felt right. Amelia was five and about to start big school, and we were happy in Kilkenny.

Jim's eyes lit up when I told him. I could tell he hoped it would be a boy. That would complete the picture.

19

Buyer Beware

IKNOW THE RECESSION HIT everyone, but I can't help but feel it hit some worse than others. In a way, I thought we had escaped it. Jim was still getting work and we were making our mortgage payments, which was the main thing. But the recession dominated the daily news: cutbacks in spending, job losses, ghost estates abandoned across the country. The banks were failing, and it felt like they were taking everyone down with them. Everything in the country slowed down, especially building work.

Jim's father's building business mainly worked on public contracts – restoring old buildings, such as convents and hospitals, often for the Health Service Executive or the Office of Public Works. So the work was still coming in, despite the downturn. But in December 2010, just before Christmas, the recession finally decided to pay us a visit; it was about to get personal. Jim came home one day looking stressed. I knew immediately. I had been fearing this for months.

'What is it?' I asked over the dinner table.

'I had a chat with Dad today,' he said.

My shoulders tightened. I knew what was coming.

'We're winding up in April.'

I tried to think of what to say. I didn't want to react emotionally. I knew this was hard for Jim. I was seven months pregnant and we were facing into Christmas time. The baby was due in February and with our two salaries we were just about coping financially.

That night when Jim and Amelia had gone to bed, I stayed up, sitting by the fire with Jim's news playing on my mind. I just sat there, listening to the silence, thinking. I looked around at what we had created: a big house – high ceilings with more rooms than we knew what to do with, and space all around us, as far as the eye could see. This is how we pictured our idyllic family life. A place in the countryside where the children could run around, a big house with plenty of room for everyone. It sounded like a dream. Too good to be true, I thought.

The pressure mounted. We were struggling every month to pay the mortgage and the bills. Every time we paid a bill, it felt like the clock started ticking for the next payment. It was relentless.

The silence of the countryside, which had once seemed peaceful, began to grate on my nerves. At night the silence felt deafening; it was lonely and isolating. I missed the suburbs and the camaraderie of living close to others. People in the village were friendly, but at night time the village seemed a long way away. It felt like we were marooned without a community. We had the nice house, but the people were missing. I put my hands on my stomach. I could feel the baby kicking; very soon the baby would be arriving. Something had to change – and quickly.

Vicky Phelan

The next morning I sent my boss an email to ask to speak to her in private. She wrote back and scheduled a meeting for that afternoon. I was nervous walking into her office. It's hard to admit to someone that things are not working out. I told her we were having difficulty paying our mortgage and that Jim was about to lose his job, that we needed to sell the house and move back to Limerick. I was due maternity leave soon, but when I came back I would need to travel in from Limerick, which would mean different working hours. Limerick was a two-hour drive from Waterford. Helen was very understanding and reassured me that we could make it work.

That night I broached the topic with Jim. 'We need to go back …'

'What?' he said, taken off-guard.

'… to Limerick. We need to go back to Limerick. None of this makes sense any more. We have a house in Limerick with half the mortgage.'

Jim looked uncomfortable.

'We're not coping, Jim.'

He knew I was right. I could tell he felt responsible. Men always do. No matter how much society moves on, there's an instinct in men, a pressure to be the provider. The recession was robbing this from hardworking men and women all over the country – the sense of pride and dignity in doing an honest day's work. I could see Jim felt robbed. He had done nothing but work hard his whole life. And suddenly that was gone. His livelihood. His sense of self. We decided to put thoughts of moving on the back burner, at least for another few weeks.

On 26 February 2011, Darragh was born. A beautiful healthy little boy, weighing 8 pounds 12 ounces. He was such a happy baby, from the very beginning. He seemed to smile from the moment he was born. I was worried my demons would return, that I'd get post-natal depression again, but so far I was feeling okay.

The months went by. Darragh was growing and changing in little ways every day, the way newborns do. He brought so much happiness to us all.

Then, in April, as we suspected, the family business had to be wound down. The extended family felt the repercussions – it was hard for everyone. Jim's father organised a redundancy settlement for Jim and his brothers, to tide them over until they found work somewhere else. It nearly broke his father financially, but he felt the responsibility of keeping the family going. The payout helped to get us through initially. But it wouldn't last long.

Every day Jim was on the phone, calling people locally, ringing anyone he knew in the trade, looking for work. It had all dried up. No one was building, and that was that. I suggested he apply for a grant to go back to college so that he could upskill and retrain. He was reticent at first. What good was college when we needed food on the table? I explained it would be better than piecemeal work. At least we would know where the next cheque was coming from. Through social welfare he could be paid a small amount every week for the duration of the four-year course. Eventually, after another round of unsuccessful phone calls, Jim agreed to give it a go. He sent in the application and was accepted onto a degree in Mobile Communications and Security at the University of Limerick, which was only a short walk from the house we owned there.

I found a school for Amelia to transfer to. She was now going into first class and she would be starting at the local Gaelscoil. We also secured a place for Darragh in the crèche around the corner from our house. It was very important that both kids were within walking distance of the house since I would have the car a lot of the time for my commute up and down to Waterford and we wouldn't be able to afford a second car. At least with a back-to-college allowance we would have a steady amount coming in every week, something to rely on. Coupled with my salary, we would just about manage.

We put the house in Kilkenny on the market, hoping some young couple would snap it up, the way we did. The weeks went by. There was some interest, a few viewings. Couples arrived, looked around, talked excitedly about what they would do with each room, why it would be perfect for them and their future family. They would leave, with promises to be in touch. And then we'd never hear from them again. No one was buying; no one *could* buy in that economic environment. So we were stuck with a house we couldn't afford.

We moved back to Limerick and found tenants who were willing to rent the house in Kilkenny, but at a very low monthly rate. It went a little way to paying the mortgage, but we were still supplementing it. Eventually, we found buyers, but had to sell for a fraction of what we had paid for it. *Caveat emptor*: buyer beware.

It was around this time that something very unexpected happened in work. After Amelia was born, I had volunteered to become the first-aider. It meant I would have the chance to attend first-aid classes. I wanted to be sure I could help Amelia if anything ever happened at home. I never thought I would have to use the skills in the office. The phone on my desk rang.

'Am I speaking to the first aid responder?'

'Yes,' I said, quite taken aback.

'We need you to come downstairs, quickly. We have a

medical emergency. It looks like an epileptic seizure, but he's not moving.'

I dropped the phone and ran down the stairs. I was feverishly trying to remember all the things I had learned in my first-aid classes. When I reached the bottom of the stairs, I saw a young man lying on the ground with a group of people gathered around him. He didn't appear to be moving.

I ran into the middle of the circle of people, and knelt beside him. I took his pulse. Nothing. I felt again, desperately hoping to feel even a faint heartbeat. I put my hands on his chest. He wasn't breathing. The boy could not have been more than twenty or twenty-one. He lay there motionless on the floor of the college hall.

As I readied myself to start doing CPR, the nurse arrived and asked me what I thought, and made her own assessment of the situation. We both started administering CPR, taking it in turns until the paramedics arrived. Even though it was clear to both of us that this young man was dead – rigor mortis was starting to set in – we kept it up because we both knew that if there was any chance of him pulling through, we needed to keep oxygen going to his brain. The crowd of onlookers knew too and silently watched on.

The ambulance arrived a few minutes later, and the paramedics took over, lifting the man onto a stretcher. I was shaking. I told them what I had found on arrival. Everything got very busy very quickly. One paramedic climbed onto the stretcher, arched over the man's body, and continued to administer CPR while the others wheeled him into the ambulance.

At that moment, all I could think of was Christophe and the sudden loss of life. Soon a family somewhere would receive a knock on the door that would shatter their world. They would have crossed that line, into pain, real pain. My heart was heavy, knowing what awaited them. Someone handed me a cup of sugary tea. 'Drink this,' she said. 'You must be in shock.'

It put everything into perspective. That night when I got home Amelia ran towards me to say hello, as she always did when I came through the door. I scooped her up in my arms and held her close. I went into the bedroom and kissed Darragh goodnight as he lay in his cot. I wished for them to always be safe in the world. At least for now, we could protect them, that was our job.

Getting into bed, I turned to Jim and said, 'We're going to be alright.' You can worry about money and bills and mortgages, but as long as your family is alive and well, that's all that ever really matters.

20

The Worst Thing

I FOUND OUT JUST HOW TRUE that is, just a few months later.

Most people when they meet me today ask me how I cope, how I keep going. What they don't realise is, cancer isn't the worst thing that has happened to me. Something much worse happened, something I still find hard to talk about.

The year was 2013. It was a cold January evening. I remember driving home from Waterford. I had been working late. I was tired and had been feeling particularly low. The post-natal depression had come back. The financial strain of our situation, and Jim's unhappiness at being made redundant, were all weighing heavily on my mind and the long commute from Limerick to Waterford was starting to take its toll. But I tried to stay strong, to be as normal as possible, especially around the kids.

When I got home, Amelia was upstairs having a bath. Darragh

was already in bed. I could see the light on in our bedroom; Jim was studying, working late as he often did.

Amelia heard my car pull up in the driveway. She called down to me. 'Mam!'

'Hi, petto. I'll come up to you now.'

She was sitting on her bed, just out of the bath, choosing something to wear.

'Will I dry your hair for you?'

'No, I'm okay, Mam. I'll do it myself.' Amelia was seven now and had started wanting to do things for herself.

I went downstairs to the kitchen while she was getting dressed. Whenever I came home late she would wait up to see me so that we could have a little chat together. I'd check her homework and we would have a cup of tea. It was our time, just us, without the boys. I knew she looked forward to it. And so did I.

A few minutes later she came bounding down the stairs. Even though it was January, she had put on a long flowing summer dress. I can still see it. She went into the sitting room. She turned on her Barbie programme and I could hear her, prancing around, twirling and dancing to the music as she always did, while I made the tea in the kitchen. To this day I cannot bear to hear that Barbie music. It reminds me of that night.

We had the fire lighting in the sitting room. I had collected firewood from Dad just a few days beforehand. We were really struggling financially, and Mam and Dad were doing anything they could to help us. Mam was always baking things for the kids and Dad would give us wood for the fire. That kind of thing.

I remember the wood was particularly dry. I remarked on it when I'd gone to pick it up. It was cracking in the fire, the way wood does when it's bone dry.

Amelia was singing along to the music on the television when a splinter escaped past the fireguard and set fire to the back of her dress. Because of her blindness in her right eye, she didn't see the flame until it had made its way all the way up her skirt. The dress was made of cotton and it had a full skirt, which was why it must have caught fire so quickly. And Amelia did the instinctive thing, that any child would do: she ran, the air fuelling the fire. She came rushing through the kitchen door screaming. I turned; all I could see were flames coming through the door, and all I could hear were her screams. Those screams. I'll never forget them. I dropped both cups of tea and they fell to the floor.

'Jim!' I shouted.

He knew from the way I was screaming that something was seriously wrong. He came running down the stairs. 'Vicky! What is it?'

'Jesus, Jim. Jesus ...'

His face went white when he saw Amelia screaming in pain and writhing on the floor. I was trying to get the dress off her. The fire was still going. Jim got down on the floor and tried to rip her clothes. His hands were burning as he pulled the material. I remember the smell of burning flesh. Amelia's and Jim's.

'What will we do?' he yelled.

He managed to rip the last shred of cloth from her skin. He scooped Amelia into his arms. Her face was wet with tears. She was white as a ghost. 'Will I put her in the bath?'

'No! No! Don't!' I screamed as he ran up the stairs with her.

'No, you'll kill her, Jim. You'll kill her if you do that. You have to keep running water on it. It has to be warm.' I don't know how I remembered that from my first-aid course, but somehow when I really needed it, that piece of information came to mind. We stood her in the bath and Jim was hosing her down, using the showerhead to keep the warm water running over her.

'Keep your arms out, petto. You're going to be okay. You're going to be okay. Mammy's here. Mammy's here.'

Her body was blistering and red raw. The doctors said afterwards that if she hadn't held her arms out at that moment they would have fused to her body and she would have had a disability. I don't know what instinct kicked in to make sure she didn't put her arms by her side.

I ran downstairs to call an ambulance. When I got to the kitchen the dress was still on fire in the middle of the floor. I grabbed a basin from the kitchen sink and threw water over it and stamped it out.

My hands were shaking as I searched for my mobile phone in the bottom of my handbag. I dialled 999. The three digits you never want to have to call for your children. I got through to the operator. 'My child has been in a serious fire incident. She needs help urgently.'

'What is your name? For our records.'

'Vicky Phelan.'

'Okay. What is the name of the person in need of assistance?'

'Amelia Phelan.'

'What is the address?'

'Carrigeen, Annacotty, Limerick.' I could barely get the words out. I couldn't believe this was happening to Amelia, that I was saying my daughter's name to the ambulance service. Suddenly

I found enormous energy. 'She has suffered severe burns to her upper body. We need help. Come as quickly as you can.'

I hung up and ran out to the neighbours' house. I banged on the door and rang the doorbell again and again. 'Joanne!' I yelled. 'Joanne! It's Vicky! It's Amelia. She's hurt.'

Joanne opened the door. 'Vicky! What is it? Is everything okay?'

'It's Amelia. She's been burned …' I couldn't say the words. I could see she knew it was serious. 'The ambulance is on the way, will you keep an eye out for it?'

And then I thought of Amelia's best friend Sinéad – her mother was a paediatric nurse and lived around the corner. I was about to run to her house.

'What is it, Vicky?' Joanne said. 'Let me do something to help.'

'Can you get Sinéad's mother? Number 30.'

'Of course. Good idea.'

Siobhán, another neighbour, had come to her door in her dressing gown. 'I'll get her,' she said, and quickly made off down the road. I went back into the house. A few minutes later I heard the sound of voices at the door and Sinéad's mother Lorna, and her husband Ian, came running up the stairs.

'That's right. Keep your arms out, Amelia. You're going to be okay,' I said, trying to comfort her.

Then came the sound of a vehicle pulling up outside and a man arrived who I recognised from Amelia's school. He was the father of one of the children in Amelia's class. He recognised me too. 'I'm the first responder,' he said. 'They've sent me out. Where is the child?' He ran upstairs with his first-aid bag. Suddenly there were a lot of people in the house.

I was shaking. My little girl was in so much pain.

'Pack a bag, Vicky. Gather some things.'

Lorna took out a bag for me. 'Tell me what to put in it, Vicky. A change of clothes. A toothbrush. You'll need it. You'll be going to Cork.'

'Cork?'

I couldn't think straight. I didn't know what she was talking about.

'Yes, they'll take Amelia to Limerick for assessment and then straight to Cork,' she said, having made her own assessment of the seriousness of the burns.

I felt like I was in a dream. More like a nightmare.

'We need to get her to the hospital,' I heard the first responder say.

We quickly made our way to his vehicle. Amelia was lying across the seat, with her head in my lap. 'It's going to be alright, petto,' I told her. 'It's going to be alright.'

We pulled out of the driveway and the siren bellowed, breaking the silence of our sleepy neighbourhood. We must have broken every red light on the way. Lorna followed us in her car. Jim had to stay behind to call my parents to come and look after Darragh.

We arrived at Limerick Regional Hospital. The doctors quickly assessed Amelia, gave her some strong painkillers, applied a burn pack and rushed us through to where the ambulance was parked and ready to go. We got in the back of the ambulance. This time Amelia could lie out on the stretcher. I tried to keep her talking, to keep her engaged. I kept asking if she was okay, or if she would like anything. I don't know how she didn't fall unconscious with the pain.

Suddenly I had the urge to be sick. The paramedic passed me a plastic bag. I vomited two or three times on the way to Cork, in between talking to Amelia and trying to calm her down. I was trying to make light of it so that she wouldn't panic. By the time we got to Cork I thought she was starting to look a little bit better. I tried to convince myself of that.

When we arrived at the hospital, she was immediately lifted out of the ambulance and her stretcher pushed through the door. Then I knew it was bad. There was a group of doctors waiting for us. The reality was hitting me again: there are too many people here for this not to be serious. We were greeted by the plastic surgeon, who tried to reassure me. 'She's in good hands, now. She's going to need to go into surgery,' he said.

'Now?' I said.

'Yes, there's no time to lose.'

Amelia could see that they were taking her away from me. She let out a scream and started crying. 'Mammy!' she wailed. I put my hand to my mouth. I couldn't believe this was happening. She didn't want to be separated. She was so scared.

'It's going to be okay, petto. Mammy's just here.'

They took her into the operating theatre. The doors closed behind them. Suddenly she was gone. They showed me to the waiting area and gave me a seat. Please just let her be alive, I thought to myself as I sat there. Please, let her live, let her live. It was like a mantra going through my head.

After what seemed like a long time, Jim came through the door. He had driven all the way down, once Darragh was safely in the care of my parents. I don't know how he had the strength to drive with all that going through his mind. I was so relieved to see him.

'Where is she?' he asked, looking worried.

'They've taken her into surgery. They said it will be some time before she's out.'

He sat down next to me. He looked like he was in shock. We waited and waited. Six hours later the plastic surgeon emerged. 'She's doing well,' he said.

'Oh thank God.' I felt like I could breathe for the first time in hours.

Jim took my hand and squeezed it tight.

The surgeon continued to talk us through the procedure. They had to move quickly so that they could clean her skin, to prepare her for the skin graft surgery so that she wouldn't get any infections. She was stable now, she was doing well, he told us.

He brought us to see her. She was in the isolation unit. There she was on the bed, wrapped up in bandages. Our little baby. She was fast asleep. I stayed beside her. The staff on the ward were very attentive. They came to check on her throughout the night.

We were at Cork University Hospital for the next five weeks. She had to have two skin grafts. It was a lot for her to take in. We tried to explain to her what had happened. She was so confused and she was in pain.

Mam and Dad brought Darragh to see us. Mam gave me a hug when she got to the ward. For the first time, I knew what she and my dad must have been feeling, waiting by my bedside in France, hoping I would recover. Now I was doing the same thing with Amelia. This time I was the mother. This was harder, somehow.

Jim stayed in the hospital too, but travelled back and forth to Limerick to check in on Darragh every few days, so that he would have some sense of normality, with at least one parent around. I knew it wasn't a good scenario for Darragh, being without us for so long; I know it affected him. But at that time, all I could focus on was Amelia getting better. Everything else would be okay. If only we could bring her home again.

Finally the day came for her to leave the hospital. We were all apprehensive about the journey. She was still covered in bandages and was very delicate. She cried a little in the car. It was hard for her to be away from the comfort and reassurance of the hospital. I tried to calm her. 'Your bedroom's all ready for you, Amelia,' I told her. 'We've made it very cosy and you'll have all your toys and books around you and Mammy and Daddy will be there. And Darragh.'

We arrived at the house. It was the first time I had been there since the night of the fire. It was a different place now. It held that memory. That night I changed her bandages. She was in tears.

'It hurts,' she said.

'I know, petto, I know. It'll be better soon.' I kissed her forehead.

She lifted her t-shirt and I began to peel off the bandages. It took all my strength not to cry when I saw her body again. Her skin was still red raw. The burns had gone all the way up her body and across her chest. 'But she's alive,' I kept telling myself. 'She's home. And she's alive.'

I went downstairs afterwards to make a cup of tea. As I walked past the sitting room, I stopped to look at where it had happened. The ash from the fire was still in the grate. That cold hard shell of a fireplace, standing like a monument to the destruction it had caused, the pain it created, with its vicious tentacles of flames.

She had nightmares for months afterwards. She often woke

in the middle of the night and would cry, like she had just had a fright. We took turns sleeping with her. When she woke, we comforted her, whispering to her or singing a gentle song, until she drifted back to sleep.

Darragh was different too. It had affected him, even though he was not yet two years old. Whenever Jim or I left the room he cried. He had a fear of us leaving him. So, when one of us was sleeping with Amelia, the other one was sleeping with Darragh. For the next few years he would very rarely sleep on his own.

We were all different after that night. Jim threw himself into his college work; it was his way of dealing with things. He became quieter too. He was never much of a talker, but after that night, he spoke less and less. He would come home in the evenings, get something to eat and go upstairs to study.

It was a lonely time. We were both suffering, but we didn't know how to talk about it. We both carried guilt, and sadness. How could this have happened in our own house? To this day it is the hardest thing to talk about. It was the worst thing, of everything. When it is your own child and you cannot make their pain go away, there is no greater pain.

Amelia grew stronger as the weeks went on. We got into a routine. I changed her bandages every night. She wouldn't let anyone else touch her or go near her, not even my mother.

I could see she was starting to get lonely, being on her own in the house all day. She missed school and her friends. So we invited her best friend, Sinéad, to come over to the house.

I was worried about how it would go. You know the way kids can say things, without meaning to. I didn't know how Sinéad would react to seeing Amelia, or how Amelia would feel by her reaction. She was going to be the first friend to see her since the accident.

That afternoon, before Sinéad arrived, I called Amelia downstairs for some juice at the kitchen table. I could see she was nervous. I decided to talk it through with her. We always do that; we talk about everything. I don't want her to think anything is off-bounds.

'Are you looking forward to seeing Sinéad?' I asked.

'Yeah ...' she said, unconvincingly.

'Anything you want to chat about?'

'No ...'

I could tell there was something on her mind.

'Why don't you show Sinéad your scars,' I said. The burns had healed up but the scars were there to stay. They would be a part of her life forever, so it was important she learned to accept her new body, scars and all. 'There's nothing to worry about. This is you now, Amelia.'

The doorbell rang and Amelia's face lit up. She missed her friends. Sinéad was at the door, with her mum. Immediately the two girls went running upstairs to Amelia's room.

Sinéad's mum, Lorna, came into the kitchen to have a cup of tea. 'How is she?' she asked.

'Getting much better,' I said.

'And how are you?'

My eyes welled up. 'It's so hard,' I said.

She nodded her head. She understood. Mothers do.

I tip-toed upstairs to check in on the girls, to see if they wanted a juice. I saw Amelia lift her t-shirt and I held my breath, waiting to see how Sinéad would react. I was so proud of her, bearing her body to her friend. Her war wounds.

A few seconds passed while Sinéad surveyed the situation,

before giving her verdict. 'Oh,' she said, 'you just look sunburned!'

Amelia smiled. I breathed a sigh of relief. She wouldn't be worried now about going back to school.

21

The Big 4-0

I T WAS 2014. DARRAGH WAS three and Amelia was eight. Somehow we had managed to move on from the fire, managed to keep going as a family. But Jim and I were more distant with each other since that night. He never spoke much about anything anymore, and I couldn't speak to him about what had happened, so we avoided talking, mostly. The children were our new focus in life. I decided to concentrate, as best I could, on the positive. Darragh was happy and Amelia was recovering well. We tried to enjoy the wonderful ordinary things that family life brings, reading stories to them, bringing them on little outings and having their friends to the house to play. Everything revolved around the children. Maybe it's because we wanted to erase the trauma of what they had experienced. We wanted good memories, to replace the bad. They were both going through big changes in their lives. We watched as Darragh turned into a toddler, showing signs of his ever-growing personality. He was adventurous, curious about everything and full of love. He had a smile that kept us going, through everything. And when he laughed, his cheeky little chuckle, he made us laugh too. He was the sunshine in every day.

Amelia was doing well in school and had made a full recovery. I was in awe of the strength she showed, to be able to continue on after all she had been through. It was hard, and it took time before she began to feel like herself again. She was scared a lot, cautious of things in a way she had never been before. We had borrowed some money to send her to counselling and it seemed to be helping her to regain her trust in things. Time will pass and her life will move on, but I know she will carry the scars – physical and mental – from that terrible accident for the rest of her days. And so will I. But we all had to be strong, because Amelia was the one who had gone through it, and despite her years, she had the fortitude to be able to pick up and keep going. So we all followed suit.

We decided to take a family trip to Galway for the June bank holiday weekend. We packed up the car with swimsuits, buckets and spades, buggies and car seats. It was filled to the brim. The kids were full of excitement.

When we arrived, we explored the city and went to the beach. Amelia built sandcastles while Darragh knocked them all down. Then off for an ice cream and back to the hotel to settle in for the night. After dinner, we put the children to bed. We were all tired from the sea air.

Jim and I had sex that night, which hadn't been happening very often. Maybe it was because we were away from home, in holiday mode. We had been growing apart since Amelia's accident. It was good to feel close again.

But afterwards, I got a terrible shock. I noticed blood coming from my vagina. I was bleeding profusely.

'What's wrong?' Jim said as I leapt to my feet.

'I'm bleeding,' I said. There was fresh angry red blood on the crisp white sheet.

Jim tried to comfort me. I went to the bathroom. It took a while for the bleeding to stop. Jim knocked on the bathroom door after a few minutes. 'Are you okay?'

'I am now,' I said, coming out, 'but I think I need to see a doctor.'

I was shaken. I had never suffered with periods. Since I was a teenager, I had been regular, every month, without question. Recently, I had noticed that I was bleeding in between my period, not a lot but what was strange was the colour of the blood – it was light pink rather than the unmistakeable dark red of a period. My periods had also become a little heavier and lasted longer. That was the first sign that something wasn't right. I had put it to the back of my mind, and wondered if it could be the onset of early menopause.

But after that incident in the hotel room, I knew I needed to get it checked out, properly. I booked a doctor's appointment the minute we got home. When I arrived at the doctor's, she was surprised to see me there without the children. I asked for a smear test. I was due one that year.

The doctor checked my chart. 'Your last smear was in 2011 and it was normal,' she said, checking her records. She wasn't unduly worried.

The nurse took the smear. 'This is a bit unusual,' she said. I was bleeding as she took it.

I'd had friends who'd had the LLETZ procedure, where pre-cancerous cells are lasered off your cervix. I worried that it might be pre-cancerous cells. Other than the bleeding and the bit of weight gain around my middle, I didn't have any other symptoms.

I was with my friend Eilish having lunch at work when the phone rang exactly four weeks later. Eilish saw my face change when I took the call.

'I have the results of your smear and I need you to come in to me,' the doctor told me.

'What are you telling me? Are you telling me there's something seriously wrong here?'

'Well, there are some high-grade changes,' she said, 'but I really do need you to come in to see me.'

I felt panicked when I put down the phone. Eilish tried to calm me. Things seemed to happen very quickly after that. The GP told me I would need to have a colposcopy. The colposcopy appointment was made for 15 July.

The consultant at the hospital gave me a local anaesthetic. I put my feet up and he started poking around. He put a dye on my cervix to see if there were pre-cancerous cells.

'What is it?' I asked.

'We won't know until we have the biopsy back,' he said.

The smell in the room brought back memories of burning flesh. It reminded me of Amelia's accident. I closed my eyes. I couldn't tell him everything that was going on in my head. Meanwhile, the noise of the laser sounded like a mechanical saw. Lasering my bits. I felt like I was being torn apart, from the inside. He gave me a prescription for very strong painkillers. When I sat down in front of his desk, he said something I really wasn't expecting. 'Are you finished having your children, Mrs Phelan?'

'Pardon?'

'Are you finished having your children?'

'Yes … I've got my two children.'

'Okay. I'm going to book you in for a hysterectomy,' he said.

'Are you telling me I've got cancer? Is there something you're not telling me?'

He reassured me that it was just a preventative measure because the changes were so high-grade and it was better to not allow these changes to develop into cancer. We would have to wait for the biopsy results to come back.

I rang Jim and told him I was ready to go home. A few minutes later he texted to say that he was in the parking lot. I walked out to him. I was waddling like a duck, with pads between my legs. I was sore and uncomfortable.

I got into the car. 'I have to have a hysterectomy.'

'What?' Jim was surprised.

'Yeah, on the first of August.'

I rang Mam to tell her the news. We started planning for the procedure. I knew people who had been laid up for six weeks after a hysterectomy.

'We have no bed downstairs,' I said to Jim, my mind going to the practicalities. We started planning how we would get a bed downstairs.

I rang Maria, my best friend, who is a nurse. 'When did he say he'd let you know about the results?' she asked.

I told her they had taken a biopsy and they would get back to me within two weeks. In the meantime, they were booking me in for a hysterectomy as a preventative measure.

'Right,' she said, 'if you don't hear anything within two or three days, you're okay.'

Because she worked in the system, she knew what the timelines tended to be. This was on Tuesday. On Thursday, the phone rang.

I remember it like it was yesterday. It was 5 p.m., and we were on our own in the house. We had asked Mam and Dad to mind the kids for the weekend so they had driven up to Limerick and had taken Amelia and Darragh back to Mooncoin earlier that morning. I was in pain a lot of the time and I was bleeding a lot after the LLETZ procedure. I needed a break.

It was a beautiful day, I'll never forget it. I was in the living room with Jim. We had the windows open and we were talking about going somewhere for a bite to eat.

I wasn't expecting this call. I saw a number flashing; it was a Limerick number. I looked at Jim and said, 'Oh Jesus.' I picked up the phone. 'Yes,' I said, 'this is Vicky Phelan.' I listened intently. The call only lasted a few minutes. 'Okay,' I said, 'thank you for telling me.'

I hung up. My face went white. 'Jesus, Jim, it's cancer.'

We just sat there, the two of us, in a daze. After a few minutes I said, 'We can't just sit here. Let's go somewhere.'

'Where do you want to go?' he said.

'I don't know … anywhere. Let's go to Killaloe.'

So we drove out to Killaloe. It's beautiful there. We parked the car looking out over the lake. We both stared out the window, into the abyss. Sitting in silence.

Eventually Jim said, 'Are you okay?'

'I don't know. I think I need a drink,' I said. We found a pub by the shore. I had a drink and it settled my nerves.

'How am I going to tell Mam and Dad?' I said, eventually. It would break their hearts. I knew it would.

We spent the weekend trying to digest the news. We waited until we drove down to collect the kids, to tell my parents in person. Jim brought the children out for a while and I stayed behind to talk to Mam and Dad. 'I have something I have to tell you,' I said.

They could tell it wasn't good news.

'I have cancer,' I said. I could see the pain in their eyes, the second I said that c-word. It's the word everyone dreads most.

I tried to console them, saying it was probably nothing to worry about, though I didn't believe my own words. 'The consultant said he could see there were parts of the tumour that he couldn't laser off. But the hysterectomy should sort that,' I said.

I had asked the consultant what would happen if the cancer wasn't contained. 'Then we would be looking at a different kind of treatment,' he'd said.

At that stage we were still planning for a hysterectomy. I wanted to be proactive. We were going to move my bed downstairs, and Mam was going to come and look after the kids until I was back on my feet.

The hospital organised an MRI scan. Two weeks later, on 29 July, Mam and Dad came up to look after the kids while Jim and I went in to get the results. The consultant told me that unfortunately the cancer had spread beyond my cervix. Once that happens the hysterectomy is off the table. He was passing me over to the oncology unit. I would be under a radiation oncologist.

Oncology. Cancer. Words I never thought I'd hear.

Sometime in late August I met my oncologist. I wouldn't be

starting treatment until 9 September, which felt like a very long time. I had to go in to the hospital to have planning scans for the radiographers to plan my radiation therapy. There were weeks of waiting where all I was thinking was: it's growing, it's growing. I had nightmares about it getting bigger and bigger. I could almost feel it growing inside of me.

It was very hard. And trying to get your head around telling people you have cancer is even worse. Everyone gets upset and you're trying not to get upset.

In the quiet moments, all I could think about were my children. Not this. Not now. Anything but this, I thought. My children needed me. After everything that had happened with Amelia, they needed a strong mother. What would happen if I died? It wasn't so much the dying that scared me – it was the thought of them trying to live without me. I was their world, and they were mine.

I received my treatment plan: five weeks of radiation and chemotherapy. The chemotherapy was on a Wednesday. There was nothing I could do, but do it. I wondered if I would be strong enough to handle it. You hear horror stories of people dealing with chemotherapy. I was scared that would be me. Sometimes the cure is worse than the disease.

Dad came with me for the first session. I could see the impact that sitting there beside his daughter in a room full of sick people was having on him, though he tried not to show it. I went in at eight thirty in the morning and wasn't finished until six in the evening when I had my radiotherapy, and then it was time to go home.

After every session, I'd come home and just go straight to bed. I felt sick and weak. The next day I would stay in bed all day. I was exhausted from the chemotherapy. They give you steroids to counteract the tiredness, but the problem with the steroids is they stop you from sleeping. Then you have to take sleeping tablets to try to get to sleep. It's a vicious circle.

I couldn't keep anything down and was eating the blandest of foods. I didn't get much of the diarrhoea – some people do. I was constantly vomiting. But I didn't lose my head of hair. That was a relief. Darragh loves to play with it, and it would have broken my heart if he'd seen me without it.

They say if you have cancer above the waist you lose your hair, and below you don't. Though I lost my pubic hair. They didn't tell me that was going to happen. People don't talk about that kind of thing. They should. It's frightening otherwise. The not speaking about it makes it worse.

The chemotherapy ward was an awful place to go; I found it very depressing. A lot of very sick people who you knew were on their way out. One day I arrived for my chemotherapy session. 'Where's Mary today?' I asked the nurse. I had been sitting beside her the last time I was here.

The nurse lowered her voice. 'She died last week.'

After a while, I stopped asking. People disappeared every week. One moment they're there, and then, they're gone. It was a grave reminder of the reality of cancer: the sheer power of what we were up against.

I looked around at the other people on the ward. They all seemed older than me, in their fifties or sixties at least. I wasn't even forty yet. What am I doing here? I thought to myself. I knew I shouldn't feel this way, but it was like I had been robbed, robbed of even those extra ten or twenty years that the others had had, cancer-free. When they were my age they were probably playing with their children or going about their lives. Here I was, sitting in a chemo chair.

After five weeks, I was given two weeks off. I was exhausted. I was spending most of the day in bed. Jim was in college, and the kids were at school. One day while lying in bed I heard the familiar clunk of post coming through the letterbox. I went downstairs to collect it. There was a letter addressed to me. The logo of the Mater Private was on the envelope.

I was about to get sick. I ran to the bathroom with the envelope in my fist. Lying on the bathroom floor, I opened it. I couldn't believe my eyes. I started crying. 'For fuck's sake!' I yelled. My last treatment was scheduled for the day of my fortieth birthday.

It felt like cancer was saying, Two fucks to you, Vicky. Your last treatment on your fortieth birthday. Happy birthday. Love, cancer.

The vindictive fucker.

I'd had enough. People told me to think of it as a positive thing – the gift of treatment. People can be full of it when they don't know what to say. I know they were just trying to look on the bright side, but sometimes life is just shit. And that's what this was.

After the two-week break, it was time to go to the Mater Private in Dublin, where they would administer the brachytherapy, internal radiation to zap or melt away anything inside my vagina that the chemotherapy and external radiation hadn't managed to kill off.

My mother came with me for the first treatment. We went to Dublin on the train. The journey was hard; I needed to go to the loo a lot. I could barely make it to the toilet I was so exhausted and out of breath. My mother took my arm and helped to guide me. This should be the other way around, I thought, I should be supporting her.

They give you a leaflet and they talk you through the brachytherapy, to prepare you. But nothing can prepare you. I had to have three sessions. They took my bloods that day. My haemoglobin count was really low, which explained the awful tiredness. I had to have a blood transfusion that night.

The chemotherapy was killing my system. I had to have three epidurals in the space of six days.

They knock you out, then they insert an applicator up your vagina while you are out cold, and this is what they attach the rods to. They wake you up, wheel you down to a radiation room, put you into a chamber on your own and attach you to the rods and radiate you.

Your insides don't look like a normal woman's insides afterwards. They melt everything. Your uterus … everything. Until there's nothing left. Then they give you these things called dilators to keep your vagina open for internal exams or if you want to have a sex life again. It is a terrible cancer to get. It takes away your sense of being a woman. It's painful to have sex, if you can ever have it again, and your body is changed, irrevocably.

After the internal radiation therapy, I had to have two more blood transfusions and a platelet transfusion. Then I had a bad reaction to the transfusion. You can actually have an allergic reaction; I never knew that before. I couldn't understand why I was so violently ill.

It was impossible to sleep that night in the hospital. I had one of those headaches – like your worst hangover, when you get a headache from vomiting.

The next morning I had to do it all again. It was like a form of torture. They wheeled me down the corridor. I couldn't stop vomiting. They had kidney trays either side of me.

The anaesthetist was lovely. Very comforting.

I said, 'Is there anything you can do for me so I won't be sick?'

She gave me stronger anti-sickness meds and left them to work before they attempted to put in the needle for the epidural. I had that done three times. It was awful.

After all of that treatment, if you can call it that, I went back home. I felt like a shadow of myself.

I usually looked forward to this time of year, with my birthday and Halloween, my favourite holiday. I had missed both. All I could think was, next year we will be able to celebrate. I was feeling very tired. I spent most mornings in bed. I would hear Jim coming in with Darragh, after Montessori, to give him his lunch and I would quickly get up. I tried to be up when the kids came home, to give them some sense of normality, and then I would lie down again for another few hours.

'Is Mammy in bed again, Dad?' I heard Darragh say one day.

That broke my heart. I still hadn't come to terms with the fact that I had cancer. I was going through the motions, doing whatever I was told to do in the hospital, in the hope that they could treat it, that they could annihilate it, this thing trying to kill me from within.

I had heard so many positive stories about people being cured. I was clinging to those. I felt sure that would be my story too. I would be one of the lucky few. I had to be.

22

Scanxiety

I WAS DREADING THE SCAN results. I tried not to think too much about it until I was in the room, but I was tense. It felt like the horse was kicking at the stable door, waiting for the chance to break out again.

It was February 2015, three months since I had finished my cancer treatment. I sat across from the oncologist. 'We have your results here,' she said, 'from your scan, last week.'

'Yes ...' I said.

She studied the scan for a moment and the document attached. 'Everything looks really good, Vicky. There is no evidence of disease,' she said eventually.

I felt a weight lift off me. It was like a wave passing over me. I reached for a tissue as the tears rolled down my cheeks.

'We'll have to keep a close eye on things. You will be seen every three months for the first two years, alternating between appointments with your gynaecologist and with me,' she told me, trying to keep my expectations in check. 'But for now, it looks good.'

When I walked out of the oncologist's room I felt like I had been given a second chance at life. I had followed the treatment plan and it seemed to have worked. At least all that torture had been worth it, in the end.

I arrived home and walked into the sitting room. I watched Amelia and Darragh playing together. The loves of my life. I took a deep breath. I was alive and I could be with my children. That was all that mattered.

The cancer was gone. I could leave it behind me now. Or at least, that's what I thought. But I soon learned, it doesn't just go away. The remnants of that awful disease move through your life, in ways you couldn't even imagine possible.

23

Love And Marriage

IT WAS ALMOST 1 A.M., well past my bedtime. Jim was on his computer. The glow of the screen seemed to fill the room. By now I was used to the noise of the keyboard tapping and the fluorescent light of the computer screen. I learned how to fall asleep through it. Jim was working on his final-year project.

This was our usual routine. Tonight was different, though. My head was full of worries. Since I had been sick, we were finding it hard to cope. Financially. Emotionally. We were staying afloat, but only barely.

I was suffering from depression again. I decided to give the anti-depressants another go. I needed something to catch me and pick me up. I felt less able for things since the cancer scare. I was shaken.

I took out my diary; it was what kept me going at times like this. I could pour my thoughts onto the page. The kids were fast asleep. The house was quiet.

I was hoping this routine would soon come to an end. Jim

had received his results the day before and he was doing very well – he was positioned to get a first in his degree. He just needed to keep up his focus for this final push, and then he would be finished. Then hopefully he would be able to get a good job and we could pull ourselves out of the financial hole we had been in for the past five years.

It was torture not being able to afford things, especially psychological help, which would have made all the difference. After everything we had been through – Amelia's accident, my cancer – we were struggling to deal with everything, emotionally. We were managing to get Amelia to counselling. That was the most important thing – to make sure she was able to cope with all she had been through. It seemed to help, and I was glad of that. I knew she carried a trauma that was deep set from the accident, and I hoped to God she would be alright, in the long run. But Jim and I hadn't recovered either and I wondered what effect that would have – was having – on our family.

It was the little things too that made it hard not to have money. Whenever friends invited me to go for lunch, I made up an excuse as to why I couldn't join them. The truth was: I couldn't afford it. Jim and I were going around in old clothes. We hadn't bought anything in years. The little money we had went towards keeping the roof over our heads, feeding us and buying clothes, shoes and activities for the children.

I wrote down the numbers in my diary, so I could see it in black and white – what was left in the bank account, and how many days were left in the month. I tried to make everything stretch as much as I could. We were waiting to find out if we had been approved for carer's benefit on social welfare – we'd be two hundred euro better off a week, which would make a huge difference to us financially going into Jim's final semester.

Lately, the pressure had been mounting, and it could be another four to six weeks before a decision was made on the carer's allowance, because of the backlog in applications.

I was starting to panic as I looked at the numbers – cold and unsympathetic – staring back at me from the page. People were so good, but I was embarrassed asking our family and friends for money. My godmother, Ann, had gifted me a thousand euro before Christmas. She could see what we were going through, and was trying to help. It really was a lifeline. We had bills to pay and Christmas was an expensive time, even when you were spending very little and trying to be careful. It would be just enough to see us through to the end of January, when we hoped the carer's allowance would kick in. But as the days and weeks passed, it was looking less likely that the allowance would come through in time, if at all.

I looked down at my hands, holding the diary. My wedding rings. I thought back to the day in St Lucia, the day Jim placed the ring on my finger, on the beach in front of the altar. I thought of the promises we made to one another. It felt like a long, long time ago. I could sell my rings, I thought, if I had to – I think I could bring myself to do it. They were the only asset we had apart from the house and the car, neither of which we could live without. It didn't make sense for the rings to be on my finger, when selling them might give us enough money to get by for another few months. I would much rather the money went towards doing things with the children than sitting on my finger. I decided that I would try and find a pawn shop in Limerick and see how much they would give me for the rings. It's a decision I knew I might regret in the future, but for now, all I could think about was how we would get through the next few months.

I rubbed my temples. My head was sore. There were so many bills to pay, I felt like I would explode with the pressure. Thank God for serotonin, I thought. My medication was keeping me calm. I knew that without it I would have been very anxious and short with the kids. The anti-depressants were somehow keeping me on an even keel; they were helping me to cope. Between the money worries and trying to keep up with work and the kids, I would be very low if it wasn't for my medication.

Amelia and Darragh had both been sick for the past two weeks. We were living between the chemist and the GP. Another expense. Poor Darragh's cough had turned into a chest infection. He's so good when he's sick, but sometimes it worries me. He can be very ill without you fully realising how sick he is, because he never makes a fuss. I can always see the change in him though, I know what to look out for and when it's time to take him to the doctor. They were both on the mend now, and that was a great relief.

I finished writing in my diary and placed it down on the bedside locker. I looked up; Jim was still engrossed in his work on the computer. I suppose it gave him a distraction – something else to think about to keep his mind off the stress of money. And after all, it could be our best hope of getting out of this trap. If only he could find a good job soon. I knew that's what he was trying to do – to find the best way out, for all of us.

I decided I would make pancakes for the kids in the morning. They'd like that – a little treat before school. I turned out the light and tried to get some sleep.

The weeks and months marched on, and somehow we managed to get by, just about. Father's Day came around. Jim still hadn't found work, but over the past three or four weeks I had noticed a change in us. Things had been a bit more relaxed between us since he'd finished college. There was a little bit more time for normal, everyday life, time to be a family together. I wondered if there might still be a chance we could rekindle something between us, enough to keep us going, after twenty years together.

'Why don't we go out this weekend?'

'What?' said Jim, certain he'd misheard me.

'We could take Eilish up on her offer of her apartment in Tramore and leave the kids with Mam and Dad. I'm sure they wouldn't mind.'

Jim shrugged, but something flashed across his eyes, a glimmer of hope maybe. I knew he liked the idea. We hadn't gone out together, just the two of us, in years.

'We could go for a bite to eat in Brooklyn in Tramore ...'

I called Eilish and Mam and made the arrangements. I opened the wardrobe and picked out something nice to wear. I hadn't got dressed up in a long, long time. I had stopped caring. But I wanted to look well, to find some old version of myself. I packed our bags and we hit the road for Mooncoin. It was like the children's second home. They thought nothing of going there for a night or two. In fact, they loved it. They were always spoilt at their grandparents' house.

When we arrived at Mam's Lyndsey was just home from work and insisted on doing my hair.

'Ah no, there's no need,' I said.

'You might as well,' she replied, 'if you're going out!'

She styled my hair and gave me a hug. 'Make sure you have a good time!' she said. 'You deserve it.'

I went into my old bedroom, where Amelia would be staying. I sat down at the mirror and let out a sigh. Here goes, I thought, unpacking my makeup. I put on my foundation, and drew my eyeliner, following the contours of my eyes. I put my lipstick on and looked at myself in the mirror. Where did this old woman come from, I wondered, looking at the photograph of me and Maria which was sitting on the table. We were so young then. So full of dreams and ideas. I had no idea then what life had in store.

'You look really nice,' Jim said as I sat into the car beside him.

I couldn't remember the last time he had given me a compliment. 'Thanks.' I blushed.

We sat at a table by the window. Jim ordered the wine. He talked about his college course, I talked about work, things we hadn't spoken about in months. He had been finding it difficult, studying instead of working. He wouldn't say it, in so many words, but I know him. He was relieved and proud to have finished it. We raised a glass to mark the end of a tough four years of studying.

Staying at Eilish's holiday apartment nearby meant that we could both have a drink and relax. I opened the door to the apartment and we got settled in.

'Gin and tonic?' Jim asked, taking the glasses out of the cabinet. He looked nervous.

'Yeah, go on,' I said.

We opened the double doors on to the balcony. It was just about warm enough to sit out, with blankets on our laps, enjoying the light of the long summer's evening. We made small talk, both wondering what would come next.

When we finished our drinks, it was beginning to get dark, and there was a cold chill in the air. We moved inside. I got ready for bed, and so did he, each going through the motions of our nightly routines. The room had two single beds; I wondered if Jim would suggest pushing them together. I went to the bathroom to brush my teeth.

When I walked back into the room, Jim was in bed. The two single beds were still standing apart with a gaping hole in the middle. I knew we could both feel the gap, the chasm, and everything it stood for, as we got under the covers in our separate beds. The sadness of it hung in the air, a deep feeling of loneliness. How you can be together and apart at the same time.

I knew Jim didn't want to hurt me. My body was different now and he was trying to protect me. But I missed him. I missed us. And as we both lay awake in the silence of the night, I knew in my heart something needed to change.

24

Getting Dark

THERE WAS ONE THING THAT was still keeping us together, something that meant more to us than anything: the children. Especially Amelia. She was still very vulnerable and she needed us. From the time she was born, Amelia's medical condition formed a big part of our lives together; it was a constant worry and concern. In a way it was the only thing we had in common anymore – minding her, and Darragh, making sure they were okay. Her condition had been stable for some time, but we knew that could change at any time, and it did, just a few months later.

It was 19 December 2016 when she came to me, squinting.

'What's wrong, Amelia?'

'I can see them, Mam.'

'See what, petto?'

'The floaters.'

'What do they look like?' I asked.

'It's all dark and cloudy and I can see three or four of them,' she said.

My blood ran cold. We had been warned that if she ever saw floaters in her eye – like little black flecks – we were to get in touch with her ophthalmologist straight away. It was a sign that she may lose her sight entirely.

It was so close to Christmas I worried we might not be able to get an appointment with her doctor. I rang the clinic in Waterford. I got through to one of the secretaries on the phone. She told me that the clinics were full. I persisted. 'Please,' I said. 'Just tell Dr Eugene Ng that it concerns a patient of his, Amelia Phelan – and that she's seeing floaters. Will you just get that message through to him, please? He'll see her. I know he will.'

Eugene phoned back a few minutes later to say that he would see Amelia as soon as we got there, if we could get in the car immediately and travel to the clinic. We made it to the hospital shortly before 5 p.m., just in time for some scans to be taken of Amelia's eyes. Eugene looked at the images from the tests, and confirmed that her condition had escalated again.

It is like a parasite that lives in the back of her eye. It can be dormant for long periods of time, and then it can strike again. Up until the age of five she was in a high-risk phase, and was on medication and under close surveillance. After the age of five, they said the chances of the issue recurring were slim, but that puberty and changing hormones might cause it to get worse. It was right on cue, as she was eleven and just entering that phase of life.

After a discussion with her infectious diseases consultant, Dr Wendy Ferguson, Amelia was sent home with some strong medication, to stop the infection from spreading. We made the decision to spend that Christmas at my parents' house; we needed the support. It also meant that we would be closer to Temple Street and Wendy, who oversaw Amelia's condition. I trusted Wendy with Amelia's life. She had been Amelia's doctor since she was six weeks old and was always available at the end of the phone if I had any worries.

We packed our things and moved to Mooncoin for Christmas. After two days, Amelia seemed to be getting an allergic reaction of some kind. She became very sick; she was vomiting and her skin was breaking out. She came down for breakfast one morning. I got a fright when I saw her. The whites of her eyes were yellow, her skin was itchy, and she had nearly scratched herself raw.

I rang Wendy. 'I don't know what to do, Wendy,' I said. 'She's reacting very badly to the medication.' I didn't want her to get worse as we moved into Christmas week, when it would be harder to find a doctor to help.

Wendy advised that Amelia should stop taking her medication as it sounded like an allergic reaction. We followed the advice, but then lived with the fear that the parasite would continue to thrive when it wasn't being medicated. Every day I worried that it would get worse and that Amelia would come down for breakfast one day unable to see, and would be blind for the rest of her life.

On St Stephen's Day, following discussions with Wendy, we started her on an alternative treatment. We watched closely, to see how she would react. She seemed to be doing okay, at first. We all returned to our routines after Christmas. It was a new year, 2017, but it did not start, or end, well for us.

I was at work, in the middle of a meeting, when I saw the

number of Amelia's school flash up on my phone. I panicked. 'I have to take this,' I said, leaving the room.

I answered the phone.

It was Aisling, one of Amelia's teachers. 'Amelia has had a seizure,' she told me, 'but she is doing okay now, and your husband Jim is here with her.'

The seizure had happened in the middle of class in front of all her friends. Jim was already at the school and was going with her in the ambulance to the hospital. She was stable, though, they reassured me.

I couldn't believe what I was hearing. I rang Jim. I could hear the sounds of the ambulance in the background. 'She's okay,' he said. 'We're on the way to the hospital.'

I knew Amelia could hear him, and he would be trying to sound calm for her sake. It was hard to know just how bad it was. 'I'll get there as fast as I can,' I told him.

I walked back into the meeting room.

'Vicky, what is it?' my colleagues asked.

I told them what had happened as I searched frantically through my handbag for my car keys. It was at times like this I cursed how far away my work was from home. They convinced me that I was in no fit state to drive, so I called Mam and Dad. They collected me straight away and drove me back up to Limerick. I felt like I was holding my breath for the entire journey.

We went straight to the hospital, through the busy A&E waiting room and into a curtained cubicle. Jim was sitting with Amelia, as she lay in bed. She was talking to him and she looked like she could see him. Thank God, I thought. I could feel the relief move through my body. I leant down and gave her a kiss on the forehead. 'Hi, petto! You've been very brave, I hear.' I gave her a smile.

Jim filled me in on the details. In the middle of class her friends, Eric and Kate, noticed that Amelia was staring into space and alerted the teacher. A few seconds later, she collapsed onto the ground and started foaming at the mouth. She was having a full tonic-clonic epileptic seizure. This had never happened before.

She was in hospital for two days. I met with her neurologist, who explained that because there were lesions on her brain from when she was in utero, she would have to go on anti-epileptic medication for a minimum of two years. Then, if she had no further seizures in that time, she would be able to come off the medication again. She wrote the prescription and discharged Amelia, who seemed to be feeling a good bit better, and back to herself, though we were keeping a very close eye on things.

We brought her home and invited two of her friends, Kate and Máire, to come over, just for a little while, to give her a bit of distraction from having been so sick. I could hear them giggling upstairs, so I left Jim to look after them while I went to the chemist to fetch her medication. I was just opening the door to the chemist when I saw Jim's number on my phone. I knew immediately something was wrong.

'Is it Amelia?' I asked, answering in a panic.

'She's just had another seizure,' he said, sounding out of breath.

I called for Ollie, our chemist, to come with me. 'Amelia is having another seizure!' I yelled.

He rushed over and we jumped into the car. When we arrived at the house Amelia was just coming out of the seizure. She was lying on her bed. She looked exhausted. Maeve, a neighbour and good friend, who is also a nurse, was sitting by her side.

Jim told me what had happened. She had been playing with

her friends when they noticed something was wrong. Kate, who had been sitting beside Amelia when she had her seizure in school, recognised the same absent look coming over Amelia's face and she ran downstairs to get Jim.

Her two friends looked frightened by what had happened. 'Everything's going to be okay,' we told them.

We brought Amelia straight to hospital again. The doctors examined her and concluded that she had developed a form of epilepsy on top of her condition. It was all linked. I couldn't believe it. I was so upset for Amelia, that she was now having to deal with another medical condition, and one which was also so unpredictable. I stroked her hand as she lay in the hospital bed. I couldn't imagine how frightening the seizure must have been for her. She was so young, and had been through so much already.

She was home again after a couple of days, and all we could do was keep a close watch on the situation and monitor her closely. She was feeling alright until about two months later, when she came to tell me the floaters had returned to her eye. Very quickly we found ourselves back with Eugene, her eye doctor. The scans confirmed that her eyesight was deteriorating more quickly.

Eugene delivered the hard truth. She needed to have an operation on her eye, otherwise she was definitely going to go blind. However, the surgery came with complications, he told us, and he wanted to get a second opinion before proceeding. He referred Amelia to a top-tier eye hospital in London for an appointment in June to see one of the world's leading ophthalmologists. 'It's what she needs,' he told us.

We didn't know how we would be able to afford to go to London, let alone the costs surrounding the appointment.

We would have to make it work, somehow, even if we had to borrow from friends and family again.

It's the hardest feeling – knowing your child needs something and not knowing how you can give it to them. I felt like a failure. She deserved better.

Just when I was starting to lose hope, someone up there answered my prayers. I think Nanny Kelly must have had something to do with it, because when we needed it most, help came, and in the most unexpected way. A few months before that, I had joined the Monaleen Cancer Support Group, not far from where I lived. I had heard about the group by chance through my local pharmacist, Ollie Halley. They offer financial assistance to people in the community suffering from cancer, and give practical help to families – lifts to and from treatment, help with cooking dinners and mowing lawns – the kind of help I would really have welcomed when I had my treatment in 2014.

I had decided to join the committee as I wanted to help the group to raise awareness about its existence among younger people in the community who, like me, were on social media. I had offered to run the Facebook page and do some promotional campaigns since it was something I was good at.

I was attending a committee meeting. Mike Reidy, the chairman, turned to me during the tea break. 'Is everything alright Vicky?' he asked. 'You don't seem yourself.' He could sense there was something wrong with me and obviously thought it was to do with my cancer.

I broke down in tears, in the middle of the meeting room. I was mortified. I explained what had been happening with Amelia, that she had to have laser surgery and that I needed to take her to see a specialist in London for a second opinion. Mike listened. I could see he really cared.

A few days later, he rang me and asked if he could call to the house to see me. I was working from home that day so I said, 'Yes, of course.' He arrived, and over a cup of tea he told me that the committee had discussed my situation and felt that because I had not been able to avail of their support when I needed it in 2014, they had decided to support me now. They were going to give me enough money to cover the cost of the trip to London, the fees for the consultant at Moorfields and the laser surgery for Amelia.

I couldn't believe what I was hearing. I cried with relief. I thanked Mike and the committee, from the bottom of my heart. They would never know how much this meant to me, how important it was, for the future of my child.

We booked the flights and the appointment and made the preparations. There was no time to lose. We could only afford for one of us to go, so I went with Amelia. I tried to make a nice weekend of it. We explored London together. I wanted it to be a nice memory for her.

We went to see a West End show and visited Madame Tussauds. It made the experience less frightening for her – there was something nice about the trip that she would remember and could tell her friends about.

The following day we went to the appointment. The surgeon told me privately about his cousin who also had toxoplasmosis. Looking at Amelia's scans, he said the condition looked very similar to his cousin's, based on the images. His cousin had gone blind. It wasn't what I wanted to hear. He told me that was a reality we may have to face, that at some point Amelia may go blind. He agreed that surgery would be her best chance at saving her sight.

I was distraught, though I pretended not to be, for Amelia's sake. I didn't want her to be frightened; I owed her that.

It was time to return home to Ireland, so we packed our bags and headed for Victoria station. As we were making our way towards the train, a fire alarm went off. Suddenly, there were armed police everywhere directing people away from the platforms.

I grabbed Amelia's hand. We stopped to listen to the announcements on the Tannoy. They were telling everyone to leave the station immediately and to follow the directions of the police and stewards. We could see people running and I started to feel panicked but tried not to let it show. We walked quickly towards the nearest police officer. He said that we had to evacuate the station and wouldn't tell me any more than that. So we did what we were told and moved quickly to the nearest exit. There were swarms of people trying to exit at the same time.

Once we were above ground I felt less afraid. I took my phone out of my pocket, to see if there was anything about the incident online. People beside me were saying it was a bomb scare. The Manchester Arena bombing had happened a few days previously, where a suicide bomber had blown himself up at an Ariana Grande concert, which was attended mostly by teenagers and their parents. Twenty-three people were killed and the UK was on high alert, anticipating another attack. We had been following the story. Amelia had been very affected by it, as she was a big fan of Ariana Grande and could relate to the teenagers at the concert. She had seen the devastation the attack had caused and was scared that something similar was happening to us. I reassured her that we were very safe, but in truth I wasn't so certain.

A few minutes later we were told it was safe to re-enter the station. Cautiously we walked back down the stairs, into the underground. There was a general feeling of unease; we suddenly felt very vulnerable. We caught the next train to Heathrow. The carriage was very quiet. Everyone was tense. When we arrived at the Aer Lingus desk I told the woman at the counter about the bomb scare at the station, and how we had missed our train. There was nothing she could do, she told me. We were too late. We had missed check-in.

'I think we might need to go and sit down for a few minutes, petto,' I said. I bought Amelia a packet of crisps and a drink and we went to find a seat. I scanned the airlines online, looking for another flight to Ireland. They were all fully booked. It was a bank holiday weekend in England.

I could feel my eyes welling up with tears. I was exhausted. It was all too much. I knew that I didn't have enough of Amelia's medication to get through another day. All I could think of was the risk that she would have an epileptic fit or that her sight would get worse. I felt like a bad mother again.

I rang Ollie, our local pharmacist, and asked him if it would be possible to get her medication in the UK, if he faxed over the prescription. He wasn't sure how straightforward it would be. I went to the pharmacy in the airport and explained the situation. There was nothing they could do, they said. They wouldn't be able to give me the medication.

Amelia gave me a hug. 'Are you okay, Mam?'

I kissed the top of her head, tears rolling down my cheeks. 'I'm fine, petto.'

'It'll be okay, Mam,' she said.

I suggested we go and get some food at the bar. I needed a drink to steady my nerves, so that I could make a plan. It was looking like we were going to be stuck in England for the weekend. I tried to think of people we knew living in London. I thought of my cousin and his wife who visited Ireland every summer; I knew them well, but I didn't have their phone number. I called my aunt in Ireland. I didn't want to worry my mother. She gave me the number. I rang, but there was no answer. They must be away for the bank holiday, I thought.

We went to the bar and ordered some food. I had a pint with my lunch. Amelia looked surprised. It was very out of character for me.

'I just need a drink, Amelia. Just one after the morning we've had,' I told her.

A man who was sitting at the bar looked up. He could see I was upset. He was wearing a Guns N' Roses t-shirt. I asked him if he was going to the concert in Slane. Jim was going with his friends, so I knew it was on.

'I am,' he said. 'How did you guess?' he joked, pointing at his t-shirt. He was Irish, as it turned out, and was travelling home for the concert. 'Is everything okay?' he asked.

'We were in a bomb scare and we missed our train and there's no plane to take us and I have no medication,' said Amelia, all at once.

He immediately offered to help. We could stay in the house he shared with his girlfriend. They would put us up for the weekend. He just needed to tell his girlfriend we were coming. It would be no problem at all, he told us.

My heart lifted at the kindness of this stranger. I thanked him profusely, though I didn't want to impose on him. At that moment I remembered that Jim had a cousin living near Heathrow. She worked for an aviation company, so I googled her name and found the company. I rang and got through to reception. Fiona was away and wouldn't be back in the office until Tuesday, they said.

I explained the situation to them. 'Please contact Fiona and tell her I am a cousin and that we are at Heathrow and my child has no medication. Tell her it's an emergency.'

A few minutes later Fiona called. She invited us to stay with her and her family and told me that she would talk to her pharmacist and make sure we got whatever medication we needed for Amelia. I trusted her.

I gave Amelia a hug. 'It's going to be okay. We're going to spend the weekend with your cousins in Ascot,' I told her. And off we went.

To this day, I am touched by the kindness we experienced. So many people were willing to help us through that situation – people we knew and people we didn't know. A little kindness goes a long, long way. It is something I have carried with me since that time.

Amelia had her surgery a short time later. It was an ordeal, especially for an eleven-year-old. She was out of school for weeks recovering, but it seemed to have been a success. We hoped that her eyesight would improve; we were monitoring it closely. We were also on high alert for seizures. We were given emergency medication called Buccolam. It was like an EpiPen for children with allergies. The doctors told us we would need to administer it if she had a seizure that went on for more than five minutes. This was crucial.

It meant that one of us had to be within five minutes of the school at all times. My work was in Waterford, so for several days a week, Jim had to be the one close by. He had just managed to get another job working as a carpenter, but this would mean he would have to give that up now. We debated it for days, but in the end, there really was no question. If our little girl needed us, we needed to be there. Simple as that. Though it meant that Jim was out of work again.

It was a stressful time. Most of all for Amelia; it was a lot to deal with at her age. I tried to make life fun for her in little ways, making sure she always had friends to play with or little outings to look forward to. But the constant worry was a big part of every day. We didn't know if she was going to recover and have a period of stability or if this was going to be her new normal. We were anxious most of the time, on high alert, in case at any moment she had a seizure or saw more floaters in her eye. We had two things to worry about now. Both conditions were unpredictable and there was no way of knowing what would trigger an episode.

Because it's such a rare condition, there is no one you can ask, no 'normal' for the doctors to use as a reference point. Everyone is different. We just had to hope that she would get better, not worse, as time went on.

Often, stressful times like this bring out the cracks in people's lives. Like fissure points, the pressure builds and builds until it can take no more. That's where I was now, cracking, near breaking point.

There was something I had to do.

25

Unspoken

I WAITED UNTIL THE CHILDREN had gone to bed. I needed to talk to my husband, in private.

We started our usual routine: Jim came down for a cup of tea, I was sitting at the kitchen table, not a word passing between us. He turned the kettle on and flicked through an old newspaper on the kitchen counter.

'Jim.'

He looked startled by the sound of my voice. Our eyes met and for a fleeting moment we felt like two people who knew each other, who cared for each other. And then it was gone again.

'We can't go on like this, Jim. We need to talk about what's happening.'

'I'm exhausted, Vicky.' Jim rubbed his hands over his face and eyes and leaned against the counter, looking away from me.

'I know. We both are. We always are. Jim, we barely speak to one another anymore …'

Finally he sat down at the table opposite me. The kettle boiled, but neither of us moved to pick it up.

'Then there's the sex, or lack of it. We have to talk about it eventually. We can't go on avoiding it. I know that you are afraid to go near me since I've had cancer, and if I'm honest, I don't think that I could ever see myself wanting sex again. It's just far too painful, and I can't get past the fact that I have had tumours down there … It's not the same anymore. None of it is.

'And this can't be good for the children, seeing us like this. I don't want them to grow up thinking that this is a normal relationship.'

For years it had gone on, barely speaking to one another, to the point where the only things we talked about were logistics, or the kids, or what needed to be paid for. It became normal, but something was always missing. It was lonely. And loneliness eats away at you from the inside. Especially when you are both still physically there. It is not from the absence of one of you, it is the absence of both of you. We weren't there with each other.

We talked it through. It felt good to talk. To really see each other again.

We made the decision to push on together as parents. That's what mattered to us both – being there for our children. We had had Amelia's accident, my cancer, and now it looked like Amelia was at high risk of losing her eyesight. I could not put my children through any more upset that a break-up would surely cause. If that meant Jim and I staying together as co-parents, then that's what we would do.

I had imagined that conversation between Jim and me for a long time. I must have played it over in my head a thousand times. In my imagination we would get upset and angry, but the conversation we had that night was neither of those things. It was all very civil. Neither of us had any fight left in us.

I went into Darragh's room and curled up on the bed next to him. He didn't wake. He was used to me coming in and sleeping beside him. As I lay on his bed I felt relief, like a weight was lifted. Relief that I had spoken my mind.

We didn't have to pretend anymore, or wonder what the other was thinking. Maybe now that we had talked about it, we would both be happier and the tension would be gone. That's what I hoped for. I didn't have to feel guilty anymore.

We had practically been living separate lives for two years. We had not kissed, let alone touched one another in all that time. I blamed myself, in a way, for getting sick. It seemed to change everything. But things had been hard before that. Since the time of Amelia's accident. We were different people, after all that we'd been through.

At least now everything was out in the open.

26

Secrets

IT WAS SEPTEMBER 2017. I sat in the waiting room, waiting to be called to see the consultant. I was there for a routine check-up. I had one every three months to keep an eye on things.

I had been there for over an hour. Every time the nurse appeared with her clipboard, I looked up, thinking I would be next. People who had arrived after me went in to their appointments and left. Still I waited.

I started to wonder if something was wrong. Why was the gynaecologist holding me back? I worried it meant he had bad news for me. I sat there until every other person had come and gone and the surgery was about to close.

'Vicky Phelan,' the nurse called from the door.

I followed her into the room; I was feeling nervous. The gynaecologist stood up to greet me and shook my hand. I lay on the table and tried to settle myself. He did the usual internal exam. It was uncomfortable, but I was getting used to them. Everything seemed okay.

We had a discussion about how I was feeling generally and if I was experiencing any symptoms. I told him I was still experiencing lower back pain, which I had been feeling for some time.

'Okay, I'm going to send you for a CT scan,' he said, 'just for completeness.'

I hadn't had a scan in a long time. I felt anxious at the idea of having one again. The appointment seemed to be drawing to a close, when he cleared his throat and said, 'There's one more thing I need to discuss with you …'

He told me that the CervicalCheck screening programme had been in touch. They had carried out an audit on smears of women who had been diagnosed with cervical cancer. My smear test, taken in 2011, had been reported as normal. On audit by CervicalCheck, however, this was felt to be an incorrect result and the audit suggested that the result of my smear was in fact in keeping with 'squamous cell carcinoma'.

There was a silence in the room as I tried to take in what he was saying. 'What are you trying to tell me?' I asked. 'That I've had cancer since 2011?' My heart rate started to quicken as I totted up the years in my head. Having cancer for six years was a very different diagnosis.

He said that this was obviously a very different result from the original and that it may have impacted on my overall treatment. He then went into detail about the limitations of screening and percentages around false negatives.

I stopped him. 'If I had cancer back in 2011, what kind of treatment would I have been looking at?' I asked him.

He told me I would have been looking at a hysterectomy instead of the chemo-radiation that I was treated with.

I was motionless for a moment, trying to absorb what was

being said. We discussed the fact that I had a three-month-old baby at the time of my smear in 2011 and I wondered how I would have felt about having a hysterectomy so soon after having a baby. Would I have coped? And then a question suddenly came to me.

'Are there other women in this situation?'

'Yes,' he told me.

I was speechless. I needed to pull back. It was too much to absorb.

'I really don't have the headspace for this at the moment,' I told him. 'My daughter needs me and I am still happy to be cancer-free so I need to park this for now. But I will come back to it when I am ready to deal with it.' And with that I left the room.

I don't know what I'm going to do about this, I thought to myself. I was in shock. Is he telling me that I have had cancer for six years, rather than four? I decided I needed to put it to rest, for the moment. There was too much going on. Amelia was the priority. I was also applying for a job promotion. The interview was coming up and we really needed the money to pay for Amelia's medical bills. I couldn't take the time to process what he was saying. I needed to concentrate on what was important; I needed to focus on Amelia.

But I would come back to it. I promised myself that. This wasn't the end of the conversation.

27

The Birthday Cycle

EILISH TOOK OUT A MAP and trailed her finger along the route – Waterford to Dungarvan.

'Forty-six kilometres,' she said, 'and a slap-up meal in Dungarvan to finish! What do you say?'

She looked at me expectantly. I could tell a lot of thought had gone into this. She was setting up a little personal challenge for both of us to mark our birthdays. It would be an achievement we could celebrate. I loved her for thinking of it; she was a very good friend. It was just what I needed, though I was a little bit daunted by the idea. I hadn't been on a bicycle in years. Maybe it was time to break out of the comfort zone.

'You're on!' I said.

'Wahoo!' Eilish yelled, throwing her arms in the air. I laughed. It's amazing the power of saying yes to things. Suddenly we both had a mission to complete together. We talked about what we would need for the journey – water bottles, crackers (Eilish would bring those), helmets (we could rent) and something to wear.

'Lycra,' she said. 'Head to toe.'

We laughed at the thought.

'Sure you only live once! And we're not over the hill yet! Well, at least not for another few days!' she said, winking at me.

I had images of us heading off in our spandex, out into the elements. Jane Fonda, eat your heart out!

A few days later we were kitting ourselves out with helmets and hopping on our rented bikes, setting off to conquer the greenway. I was a little unsteady at first as I tried to get my bearings. Once I found my balance I pedalled faster, picking up speed. I could feel the wind in my hair as the world went by.

It was a beautiful autumn day. The leaves still clinging to the trees were in their evening wear – sultry red – flittering in the breeze, the last hurrah before their fall. Looking down at their fellow leaves, crumpled and brown on the ground, becoming part of the soil once more.

We followed an old railway track, twisting and turning through the countryside. We went over viaducts and under bridges and hugged the shore of the wild Atlantic ocean. As I cycled I found myself short of breath and panting. I made excuses to stop – to tighten my shoelaces, or to take a moment to look at the view. I made a mental note that I must start going to the gym to use the exercise bike. It must be drawing on different muscles, I thought.

'Nearly there!' Eilish encouraged me. 'What will we have to eat in the Tannery?'

The thought of delicious hot food and a glass of wine whet my appetite and spurred me on, propelling me towards Dungarvan. I had driven along that route many times before, but it was different to cycle it. I was taking in every turn, every bend in the road and every incline – especially the inclines. The view was beautiful. When I saw the sea, I knew we were getting close.

'Welcome to Dungarvan!' yelled Eilish as she free-wheeled down the hill.

I wasn't far behind her. As we neared the outskirts and then made our way through the town, I felt an enormous sense of achievement. There's something about traversing land. It's the explorer in each of us that feels the need to have seen it for ourselves – to have set foot in a place and travelled the distance. I thought of Eilish's finger trailing the route along the map – to think that we had covered all that ground and made it to our final destination. For experienced cyclists, it was nothing. But to us it was a mission, accomplished. We reached our hotel, cycling all the way to the front door.

'We did it!' said Eilish as we high-fived in celebration.

We went upstairs to get ready, and planned to meet for dinner at seven. I did some stretches in the hotel room. I loved the feeling of tired muscles, as though my body was thanking me for a healthy day's exercise. I stepped into the bath, lay back and closed my eyes as the hot water enveloped me.

I decided it was a day to dress up a little. My forty-third birthday. Hard to believe. And Eilish's fifty-ninth birthday.

Our meal was lovely. The waiters pulled out all the stops, and spoilt us for our birthdays.

We made a toast, 'to life!', as our glasses clinked.

I went to bed that night feeling very lucky. Lucky to have friends like Eilish. 'Forty-three might not be so bad!' I thought to myself. Little did I know how much my life was about to change.

28

Beneath The Surface

A FEW WEEKS LATER, IN mid-November, I went for the CT scan.

I felt like I was being photocopied. I dreaded to think what might be going on beneath the surface of my skin. Was the cancer back? What could they see? Had it been in my system for longer than I knew? It was all I could think about. It would be a few days before I'd know for sure.

I was given an appointment to see my gynaecologist for the results, and before I knew it, I was back in his office. This time there was no waiting around. He brought me straight in and said that, unfortunately, it was not good news. He explained that I had a large tumour, almost 10 centimetres, which was made up of five tumours on my para-aortic lymph nodes. They formed a 10-centimetre mass encircling my aorta.

Tumours – the word sent a shiver down my spine. How could it be? I had no symptoms other than lower back pain. I was not bleeding and I felt relatively good. I was tired, but I'd had a stressful year with Amelia's illness. I didn't feel like I had cancer.

I was sitting there trying to understand what this meant. The next bit, I did understand: he told me there was nothing he could do for me – no surgical options – so he was sending me back to my radiation oncologist, to see what oncology could do. Back. That's the word I heard most. Oncology. Back. Words I never wanted to hear again.

In the meantime, I'd be sent for a PET scan to get a clearer picture. A PET scan is a more detailed scan which shows up any smaller tumours, if there are any. More tumours. The thought terrified me.

I don't remember the drive home. I told Jim about the scan and what the doctor had said. I could see the worry in his face. I wanted to say, 'It'll be okay, Jim,' but I couldn't because I didn't know that it would be.

I was scared this time, really scared. I didn't want to worry my parents over Christmas.

I called Susan and asked her to come with me instead. Susan had accompanied me and Jim for my PET scan when I was first diagnosed so it felt natural to me that I would ask her to come with me for this one. I needed my friend.

I went for the scan on 11 December. I felt like I was walking through life in a daze. That week in work, I was forgetting things; I was absent-minded. I confided in some of my close friends there, Eilish and Geraldine. 'My cancer is back,' I told them. I couldn't believe those words were coming out of my mouth. It was my worst fear come true. I needed to talk about it with someone.

I decided not to tell my family. I wasn't sick and I didn't look any different than I did before I got the news, so they wouldn't be any the wiser. I didn't want to ruin Christmas for them all; I couldn't bear the idea of everyone being worried about me. If this was potentially going to be my last Christmas, I wanted it to be a good one. Memorable for all the right reasons.

Christmas Day came around very quickly. I was glad I hadn't said anything. The kids were at the age where they could really enjoy it. On Christmas morning, I could sense the excitement in the air. We kept the family tradition going; we locked the sitting room door, with all the presents under the tree.

'C'mon, Dad!' Amelia called from downstairs.

Jim kept up the game of delaying, until they could wait no longer. 'Okay, okay! Let's see if Santa has come!' he said, finally giving in. He turned the key slowly and Darragh and Amelia burst into the room. I watched Amelia – the joy she got out of the magic of it all. It's what keeps us all going, isn't it, I thought. Magic.

I wish it was real, I thought. Then we would magic cancer away. I tried not to think about the hospital. I wanted to compartmentalise it so that I could really be present with the kids. I wanted them to have good memories of Christmas time, like I did.

It was 29 December, one of those quiet days between Christmas and New Year, when I saw the hospital number appear on my phone. I immediately felt anxious. The call was brief. The oncologist wanted me to come in on 12 January. I asked if they had any news about the PET scan. She said she'd prefer to discuss it in person, that we could talk about treatment options then.

I put down the phone. It was time to tell Mam and Dad. 'The cancer's back, Mam,' I said. There was no other way of saying it. You couldn't sugarcoat cancer.

'Vicky, what do you mean? It can't be. You look so well.'

'I know, Mam. And I feel well … that's the strangest part of it all.'

It's a silent killer, cancer. Not only is it lethal, it's sneaky too. It creeps through you, without giving you a sign, until it's too late. At least other illnesses have the decency to tell you they're there. Not cancer. It plays by its own rules.

Dad came into the room. He could see Mam was upset. We were both very quiet. 'What's wrong?' he asked.

'It's back, John …' Mam said, unable to look at him.

Dad knew immediately what she meant. I could tell by the look in his eyes. In his mind he was suddenly back in the chemotherapy ward. 'No … Vicky, it isn't, is it?'

I nodded.

He walked across the room and put his arms around me. He made me feel safe, like only a father can.

I went to the oncology appointment, 12 January 2018 – a date engraved in my memory, forever. Mam came with me, and Amelia.

This brings us back to the beginning of this story – to the day I was told I had twelve months to live. I left the hospital that day feeling shell-shocked.

Though I was relieved Amelia's appointment with her neurologist had gone well. She seemed to be stable these days. I couldn't imagine not being there for her, if she took another turn. What happens to her next year, if she doesn't have her mammy? The thought frightened me.

When I woke the next morning the dawn was just breaking. The light coming through the window had new meaning for me now. My days were numbered. How many more mornings would I experience?

I made a decision there and then that I would do anything I could to stay alive. The horse had finally cornered me. At some point, I thought, there comes a time when you can't run away anymore, when you have to turn to face the horse. Meet it head-on, and say, 'I am not afraid.' That time was now.

There had to be another way to stay alive. And I was going to find it. Even if it took every last bit of me. I knew if I went back on chemo, I wouldn't be able to handle it. My body would collapse under the sheer weight of all that treatment. It works for some people, but I knew it wasn't working for me. I had started out with a 4-centimetre tumour and had done what I was told and had taken everything that was thrown at me and it hadn't worked. Here I was now with a 10-centimetre tumour mass and a terminal diagnosis.

There had to be another way.

At my next appointment, I insisted on a biopsy. I wanted to know exactly what I was dealing with, so that I could make the right decision for me. I was tired of blindly following their 'treatment' plans.

29

A Clue

MY APPOINTMENT FOR THE BIOPSY was one week later, 19 January. Mam insisted on coming with me. I was glad she was there. We arrived in the hospital for 8.30 in the morning and checked in at admissions. 'Take a seat,' said the woman behind the desk.

Once I had been admitted, we were sent up to a ward. There was a shortage of beds, so they directed me to a treatment room to wait until a bed became available. Hours went by, as we sat there, waiting for my name to be called. The nurse came and asked me to step on to the weighing scales. She scribbled some notes on my file and placed it on the desk beside me.

When she left the room I looked over at the file. I wondered what was inside it. Thoughts of the conversation with my gynaecologist were going through my mind. I needed to know if there was anything about the audit in my file. Now that I knew my cancer was back, I wanted to know more about what had happened. Once I started treatment again, I wouldn't have the energy to do anything about it.

I picked up the file and started skimming through the pages, all the records of the various medications and scans. And then something caught my eye. The hairs on the back of my neck stood up. It was a report that seemed to be about the audit.

Mam knew straight away by my expression. 'What's wrong?' she said.

'Something's not right here.'

I noticed at the very bottom of the page, in tiny print it said 'page 2 of 2'.

'There's a page missing,' I said.

'What are you talking about? It's probably just a cover page,' said Mam.

'Yes, but to *whom* and *when* was this report sent?'

I knew something wasn't right. I took out my phone and started taking photos of the document and anything else on my file relating to my smear history and CervicalCheck.

The nurse was coming back. I quickly put the file back on the table.

It was time to go for the biopsy. The nurse asked me if I was ready. A bit rattled, I said, 'Yes,' and she led the way. Walking through the hospital, I felt a sense of unease, like I couldn't trust the system. I kept replaying the conversation about the audit. What had they known that they hadn't told me? These thoughts played over and over again in my mind as I lay on the operating table looking up through the bright light at the medical team in their masks, as they removed a piece of my tumour.

*

I had no time to lose. As soon as I was back home, I took out my laptop and started researching. I wanted to be armed with information and ready for my appointment with my new oncologist. I feared that all he would offer me was palliative chemo. I searched for ways that recurrent cervical cancer was being treated around the world.

I was determined that I would find something, but the more I read, the more I realised how poor the outlook was. I tried not to let the information sink in. Perhaps I was in denial, but I was sure there had to be some option out there. I pushed aside the fear and panic and kept looking.

And then I found a clinical trial in the US that appeared to be having some success. It was based in Maryland. I read through the articles and research papers on the work they were doing. I trawled through the internet, looking at trials and hospitals across the world, but this one seemed the best fit for me, for the kind of cancer I had. I emailed the clinic immediately to put myself forward for the trial. This was my only option, I thought. I'm not doing chemotherapy again. This had to work. Everything depended on it.

The trial was using a drug called Pembrolizumab (Pembro). I put the name of the drug into the search bar and followed the trail of research papers and medical journals. I found that this drug was being used for a number of cancers in Ireland, but not for cervical cancer. It was also being manufactured by a company who had a huge presence in Ireland. I had to find out where I had to go to be able to access the drug and what I needed to do to get on it. If I could get to the source, I felt sure I would find a way to get access to it.

I did some digging. It turned out it was not that easy.

You could get it in America as they were a bit ahead of

us over there, but it was still not licensed in Ireland for most cancers, including cervical cancer, and probably wouldn't be for another few years.

I found out that the problem lay in the fact that I did not have private health insurance. I was being treated as a public patient. And so, for an oncologist to prescribe Pembro for me, 'off-label', as they call it, they would have to make an application to the medical board of the hospital. I discovered that, with Pembro, the pharmaceutical companies worked closely with a number of oncologists.

I managed to find out the names of two oncologists who were prescribing Pembro, and I could try to get referred to them. Though I knew that even if I managed to get one of them to prescribe it for me, I would probably have to pay for the drug myself.

It wasn't going to be as simple as I had thought. I had imagined that somewhere in Ireland there was a building where the drug I needed to stay alive was being stored, that they could somehow open a vault and let me in. The thought of it made me furious. And then it made me determined – determined to find an oncologist to prescribe it to me, and to somehow find the money to pay for it.

I searched for Dr David Fennelly and found his number online. I contacted his office, but was met by another brick wall. They said there was nothing they could do. I needed to be a patient of Dr Fennelly's for them to advise me.

'How do I become a patient?' I asked.

'Well, it doesn't really work like that,' they said. 'You have to get a referral.'

'Then that's what I'll do,' I said.

I knew my consultant in Limerick would not be impressed

with my request to change doctors. I didn't care anymore. I needed another option and all they were offering me was palliative chemotherapy. A death sentence, as far as I was concerned.

I needed a chance. I needed hope. Whatever form that came in. And I needed it quickly. I printed everything off and prepared a list of questions.

30

It Takes A Village

'EVERYONE'S TALKING ABOUT IT,' said Lyndsey over the phone. 'They all want to help.'

'Help with what?' I asked, trying to keep up.

'Help get you to America,' she said. 'People are coming into the salon every day asking how they can help. Some have left money in a jar. I tried to tell them not to, but they insisted.'

I couldn't believe it. Though I always knew Lyndsey would be my biggest advocate. No doubt she had been trying to find a way to help me. She knew everyone in Waterford, and they knew her. Her hair and makeup salon, Queen, was always busy with people coming and going. Word had spread about my diagnosis, and my plan to go to America.

I smiled. 'Thanks,' I said.

'There's no need to thank me,' she said, 'but I do have an idea …'

She suggested I open up a GoFundMe page – something a friend of hers had recommended. It was a way of fundraising online, a platform where people could give support, she explained.

'It's worth a go, I suppose,' I said, hesitantly. 'But is it not a bit ...' I felt embarrassed about the idea of asking for money.

'Look, Vicky,' said Lyndsey, 'people really want to do something, they just don't have a way to do it. It could make all the difference to you getting to America.'

That night I sat down at my laptop and researched setting up a GoFundMe page. The website asked me to answer the question: 'Who am I and why am I fundraising?' I wrote a synopsis as best I could.

My name is Vicky. I am 43 years old. I am married to Jim and we have two children: Amelia, 12 and Darragh, 7. I was diagnosed with cervical cancer in July 2014 and underwent an aggressive regime of radiation and chemotherapy over a 5-week period. I have had almost three years cancer-free until I had a routine scan in November 2017 which showed a large mass of lymph nodes attached to my aorta which is inoperable. Because I have already received the maximum dose of radiation, I cannot have more radiation. And so, my oncologists are only offering me palliative treatment. I have been given 12 months at most with chemotherapy treatment and 6 months without treatment.

I simply do not accept this prognosis and I am fighting with everything that I have in my power to live. I am researching the clinical trials and alternative treatments and juicing, supplementing and following a strict alkaline diet at the moment to try to stop my cancer from spreading while I wait to be accepted onto a suitable trial. At the moment, I am waiting to find out if I will be accepted onto a clinical trial in Maryland, USA. This trial is my best chance of surviving. If I get accepted, I will be hoping to fly to the States in March.

I have fantastic family and friends who are doing everything within their power to help me out but we cannot do this alone. Neither I nor my family have enough funds to cover my treatment abroad which will probably run into hundreds of thousands.

And so, I am pleading with everyone who takes time to read my story to please donate whatever you can even if it's only ten euro to give me a fighting chance to watch my children grow up and enjoy the simple things in life that we all take for granted until we are faced with not being around to enjoy the little things.

All I am asking for is a chance.

Thank you for clicking into my GoFundMe page,

Vicky

Xxx

I read over it again and again. Here goes nothing, I thought, and pressed the 'upload' button. Later that evening I sent the link to Lyndsey. 'This okay?' I asked.

'Perfect!' she replied.

A few days later, , Lyndsey sent me a text: *Wow! It's really working!*

I rang her straight away. 'What do you mean?' I asked.

'The GoFundMe page. It's gaining a lot of traction. It's fantastic! America, here you come!'

I loved her so much in that moment. The way I do all the time. But it was just so typical of her to get behind me like that.

I hurried to the computer and logged on to the site. I could hardly believe it. Donations from people across the country – names I recognised, names I didn't recognise, and messages of support.

If I was to be treated in Ireland, or if I was accepted onto the trial in America, both would be expensive. It was such a relief to see the support coming through. Maybe this would be possible, after all.

31

The Battleground

I LOOKED AT THE PHOTOS I had taken of my medical file.
I studied them, trying to make sense of it all. I couldn't work
out exactly what had happened, but I knew something wasn't
quite right.

I needed to find a lawyer, and fast. I set to work, researching
the best medical negligence solicitors in Ireland. I read articles
about the cases they had covered. I whittled it down to just two
firms, and rang the first one on my list. A woman on reception
answered. She sounded dismissive, like she didn't have much
time. She told me to write to the firm via email. It felt like she
just wanted to get me off the phone.

I jotted down the email address, then rang the other, smaller
firm. The reaction was completely different. The woman who
answered the phone wanted to hear why I was calling. She
took notes and sounded genuinely interested. She asked when I
would be available to come in to meet with Cian O'Carroll, the
solicitor. She asked me to send an email outlining the situation

and to attach copies of any documents from my file that I felt would help Cian to decide whether or not I had a case. We arranged to meet. I had a good feeling about this. Most of my decisions in life are made on gut instinct and this one was no different.

When I arrived at the solicitor's office I was met by Cian O'Carroll and Siobhan Ryan. We sat for the next hour talking through what had happened to me, bit by bit. I showed them the photographs of the papers I'd seen in the hospital and repeated the conversation that the gynaecologist had had with me, the fact that if my cancer had been caught in 2011, I may have been cured by a hysterectomy, but now, after intensive chemotherapy and brachytherapy, I was facing a terminal diagnosis. They listened intently and took notes through the whole conversation. They asked me how I felt about it all and what I wanted to come out of it. I felt listened to.

When the conversation was over, Cian looked me in the eye and said, 'Vicky, we're so sorry for what has happened to you. We're sorry you had to go through this. Let's try and make this right.'

I felt a flood of emotions. They were the first people to ever say sorry. It was the first time I'd heard the words. 'I need to know the truth,' I said. 'Before I die. I need to know what happened and why. I need to know why I won't get to see my kids grow up.'

They nodded solemnly. And like that, we became a team. They took on the investigation, examined the evidence, and decided that, yes, we had a strong case. It had been known the cancer diagnosis had been delayed by the way the slide was read, and I hadn't been told. They had *known* this information for three years.

It went from a treatable cancer, to a terminal cancer. I was going to die, but it could have been prevented. I could not imagine a greater injustice. I felt like an innocent person being sent to death row, given my last meal and told to swallow it.

We decided to go ahead and take legal action. It felt like the right thing to do. I needed answers. How and why this had happened was a mystery, but someone out there knew, and we needed to find them.

We had no idea then just how big a case this would be – what would unfold in the weeks to come and how many lives would be affected by our decision. Nor could we have known just how big a battle we would have on our hands, or that this very case would shake the country to its core.

It was just two and a half weeks since that dreaded appointment where I was told my cancer was terminal. In that time, somehow I had managed to get a biopsy, apply for a clinical trial in America, find a lawyer, set up a GoFundMe page and investigate how to access the newest drugs available. I was not prepared to waste a minute of precious time.

Now I found myself back in that familiar position: sitting opposite someone at a desk. But this time it was different, this time I felt empowered. I had my own plan of action, my own questions.

The oncologist told me that my biopsy confirmed that the cancer was a recurrence of my previous cancer, and not a new cancer. This was bad news. It meant the cancer was spreading, and the treatment options were fewer.

He was like a politician, with the same answer to everything I asked him.

'This is all we can offer you here.' He was talking about chemotherapy.

I felt as though I was drowning, that he was watching me drown. I was almost frantic. 'Surely there are clinical trials that I could try.'

He repeated his mantra. 'This is all we can offer you here.'

'And what about new drugs, like Pembrolizumab? Could I get access to that here?'

He told me that the drug was not licensed for cervical cancer patients.

'Well then, I want a referral to Dr David Fennelly at St Vincent's Hospital in Dublin. He prescribes this drug and I want a referral to see him for a second opinion.'

I refused to leave until the referral letter was written and signed. Eventually, I got it.

Ten days later, my phone rang. It was Mary, Dr Fennelly's secretary, with an appointment for 12 February. I was relieved. Now that I had taken control of my own treatment, I had no safety net, I only had myself to rely on. I knew that I needed to get on some kind of medication soon. By now, I'd had to give up work, which meant I could at least devote whatever energy I had to the pursuit.

'I need this drug,' I said, bluntly. 'I really need it.' I was sitting opposite Dr Fennelly outlining my case. I told him what I had been through with the chemo and brachytherapy treatments. He listened intently.

'You must have a lot of people who tell you these stories,' I said. 'I know you must. But this is my last chance. I need to try this drug.'

He told me that the drug was not licensed for use with cervical cancer patients in Europe. I could sense his frustration.

My heart fell. This was not what I was expecting. Another closed door. I pushed harder. 'But I am willing to pay for the drug myself. I know that you will need to get approval from the hospital board. I will sign whatever waiver you put in front of me – just give me a chance. That's all I'm asking,' I pleaded.

'The cost of this drug is very high,' he said, looking concerned.

'How much is it?' I asked. 'I've been fundraising.'

'It can be anywhere between six thousand and eight thousand euro per infusion. And you would need to get an infusion every three weeks.'

I sat back in my chair. It was a lot of money. More than we could ever afford. I thought of the fundraising page and the messages of support. Maybe it would be possible, just for a little while. 'It's worth a try,' I said, thinking it could be a stopgap – something to keep me going until I was accepted onto the trial in Maryland.

He said he would talk to the powers that be, and do his best to get it, but warned me that the answer would most likely be no.

That night I contacted my local TD, Kieran O'Donnell, who had offered to help. I explained my situation to him; perhaps there was a political answer to this, I thought. I also got in touch with the pharmaceutical company and appealed to them to intervene with the hospital and the hospital's insurers to get me on the drug. I was determined to try every avenue. I begged like I'd never begged before. But still, nothing. I was losing strength, waiting every day for some sign of hope.

I jumped every time the phone rang. I was starting to panic. I sent another email to the research nurse at the National Institutes of Health (NIH), who ran the trial in Maryland. I hadn't heard back from them. I was starting to think that America was really my only option. I wasn't having any luck in Ireland, but I still hadn't been accepted onto the Maryland trial either. I was in limbo. No solid options except palliative chemo.

What if I had made the wrong decision?

I thought back to my days in the infusion suite. I could clearly see the faces of the people sitting side by side in chairs connected to the chemotherapy machines, trying to go about their everyday lives, to keep some semblance of normality – reading the newspaper or talking to a visitor – trying to ignore the beep and hiss of the machine beside them connected to their veins. Like a life source. Only instead of air and water, it was filled with chemicals. In my mind I walked down through the ward. I saw the man with red flushed cheeks who always had time to chat, the old woman who looked so neat and ladylike, as she did the crossword puzzle, the younger man with his two daughters sitting by his side, talking and laughing, all the while trying to keep life going in the face of this awful disease without a cure. The only option: a chemical that eats away at your body until you can't stand it anymore. Until you become a scarecrow.

I wondered where those people were now, those faces I had come to know. They were frozen in time in my mind, forever sitting in those chairs. But time doesn't freeze, no matter how hard you try to make it. It thaws and melts and continues to drip by relentlessly.

32

Making The Case

W E SET TO WORK IMMEDIATELY to put a case together. We had decided to sue the HSE and the lab, Clinical Pathology Laboratories (CPL) involved in the screening. It can often take a long time to secure a court date, but the lawyers were hopeful of getting one in May. It was only a few months away, but I wondered if I would still be alive by then. I still wasn't on any medication – the cancer was growing, and I was getting sicker.

Then word came through that we had been granted a court date for 19 April. We were delighted. Ordinarily a case like this would take at least two or three years to come to court, often longer. Because I had a diagnosis of terminal cancer with a dire prognosis, my lawyers were able to ask the court for a hugely truncated process in terms of time. The courts usually try to accommodate this for urgent cases, so they had granted us a date that was just a few weeks away.

All the same work had to be done in preparing the evidence,

documenting the harm and exchanging the usual sequence of court documents, called 'pleadings', but all in the space of a few weeks. We needed to move fast.

There was still no certainty that I would survive, or if I would be in a fit state by then. We had to have a lot of tough conversations around what would happen if we went to court.

'I'm going to have to ask you to do something, and it's not going to be easy,' Cian said to me one day. 'But we have to put Jim down as a named plaintiff, in case you die.'

I understood, though it was hard to hear.

'If Jim is a named plaintiff, then we will be able to get a settlement for your family.'

I found those conversations difficult, but for Jim they were impossible. I had to have them privately with him first so that he didn't feel under pressure from the lawyers. Cian understood.

Because of my terminal diagnosis, the case was a type of hybrid action – part medical negligence/personal injury and part what is called a 'wrongful death' action, claiming not only for the pain and suffering and care costs, but also for the dependency losses of my family which includes loss of earnings, and future care costs.

We had to have all those personal conversations before the case was filed, and there was a lot to do to prepare for the trial. I had to go to a psychiatrist, and to different kinds of assessors, and a nurse had to come to my home. They needed to gather information about every aspect of my life: my work, my health, my family, my plans for the future. Cian and Siobhan were organising all the meetings, trying to spread them out, as they knew how much each appointment took out of me. For every assessment I had, I had to have two appointments: one that was for our side of the argument, and another sent by the defendants, who were also building their case against me.

Psychologically, it was difficult knowing that one professional was there to gather information that may support my case, and another to get information for the opposition, who would make a case against me, and yet I had to engage with both. The same circumstances would be used to make two different arguments.

I started to go downhill very fast. I was against the clock. With every day and week that passed, I moved closer to the six-month mark. If the consultant was right, at this rate I had just a few months to live. At night when I closed my eyes I imagined my cancer growing inside me. Left untreated, it would continue to grow.

We had to buy a recliner chair for me to sleep on downstairs as I could no longer sleep in my bed. We used some of the funds that had been raised from the GoFundMe page. Lying down had become unbearable, there was too much of a stretch on my tumours, which were now pushing out through my abdomen, and so I slept, or tried to, on the recliner in the sitting room.

Our home was changing. I was spending more time downstairs. 'If you get to a stage where you're really ill you won't be able to get up those stairs,' was what everyone was telling me.

Hearing things like that makes it very real. At the time I wasn't allowing my mind to go to that place, but at all the appointments they were talking about me dying, and providing for the children *when* I was gone. It's not if. It's all when. When. When.

I was using every ounce of energy I had left to complete my application for Maryland. The process for applying to the clinical trial was a lot more complicated than I had envisaged. They requested all my medical records, and images from my scans. As my solicitors, Cian and Siobhan were able to request all of my records to be sent by the hospital. I can't imagine how long it would have taken otherwise – I would have had to get all the information through a freedom of information request. I compiled everything I needed. I filled in the paperwork, of which there was a lot, and submitted my application for the trial. I gave it everything I had. This was my best hope of survival. I clicked the 'send' button, and waited for a reply.

A few days later, my phone rang. It was a call I really wasn't expecting – a researcher from RTÉ radio. I was confused. How did RTÉ know about me?

'We're calling about the email we received from your brother,' they said.

'What email?' I asked.

They explained that my brother Jonnie had sent them an email, telling them about me and everything I had been through. They wanted to know if I would come on air to talk about why I was fundraising.

By now, the fundraising page had raised over a hundred thousand euro. I was a little taken aback. I hadn't been expecting anyone outside of friends and family to take any notice of the fundraiser.

I had to think about it. I wasn't sure about speaking openly about something so personal. But on the other hand, it could be my only chance to get to America. What did I have to lose? I called back and agreed to come on air. A few days later, Lyndsey and I found ourselves in the RTÉ studios in Donnybrook.

They ushered us through to a seating area and Neil, a young researcher, offered us a cup of tea. The open-plan office was busy, with phones ringing and interviews taking place, people dashing this way and that, and lots of activity. It's incredible, I thought, how different some working environments can be. It was the kind of place I would have loved to work in when I was younger. Researching for a living. It seemed like the dream job.

The Ray D'Arcy Show was playing on the radio beside me. I heard him say my name as he told the audience what was coming up next. I felt my stomach lurch and my mouth go dry.

They went to an ad break, and Ray walked out of the studio. 'Hello, Vicky,' he said. 'It's lovely to meet you. Thank you for coming in to talk to me today.'

Neil, the researcher, asked me to follow him to the studio. Lyndsey was directed into the control room, where she listened to the show with Ray's producer and team.

I sat at the microphone. Ray was chatty and immediately put me at ease. I hadn't been feeling well so I was a bit out of sorts. I couldn't tell if I was nervous or nauseous. Or maybe both. It was my first time on the radio.

The red light went on and we were live. Ray welcomed me to the studio on air and gave a bit of my background story by reading Jonnie's email aloud, which almost had me in tears.

The email read:

Hi Ray

I am writing to you in hope that you could do me a huge favour and bring the plight of my eldest sister to your listeners. Her name is Vicky Phelan. She is 43 years old and the mother to 2 amazing children. In 2014 Vicky was diagnosed with cervical cancer. She underwent 5 weeks of aggressive chemotherapy and radiation treatment. This resulted in her being cancer-free for almost 3 years.

Sadly for Vicky, she received terrible news back in November when a routine scan revealed her cancer had returned in her lymph nodes, including a mass close to her aorta, which is inoperable. Vicky has basically been offered palliative treatment, 12 months with chemotherapy or 6 months without.

I would just like you to know that Vicky is a fighter and always has been. Vicky has battled through several things in her lifetime, of which I won't get into at this moment in time. But all I can tell you about her is that she is someone I am so proud of and to see her resilience even in the face of such news is hard to comprehend. It is gut-wrenchingly difficult to have to watch your sister once again face a mountainous battle, having dealt with many before. But, as I said, she always dusts herself down and faces into it. She truly is a one-of-a-kind in my eyes and I want and need my eldest sister in my life.

Vicky has done her research on this and there is a trial in Maryland USA that she hopes to get onto. If anyone has seen the documentary *First in Human*, they will know the hospital to which she is trying to gain access. Amazing work is being done in the treatment of cancer, and all diseases. If she is successful in this, the cost of her care will probably run into the hundreds of thousands. And this is where I hope your listeners can help. I have attached a link to Vicky's GoFundMe page. We would be eternally grateful if people could donate anything they possibly could to help in the fundraising. It is going to be a long road for Vicky but we believe there is hope at the end of the tunnel with the treatment on offer.

I love my sister dearly as do all my family and her friends and of course her 2 beautiful children. They above all need their 'mammy'. All we want is a little *hope* for Vicky and with every small donation it adds to that hope. I hope that you can read this out to your listeners and I hope that people can find it in their hearts to donate anything they possibly can. I hope to return to you with a story of great hope that my sister faced this and came out the other side. If there is one thing I know and have come to learn over the past while, it is that we as a nation really help each other out when the chips are down. People will rally around you when times get tough. And this is what I am hoping for. Please rally around for my sister. She deserves a better shot at life ...

Hope is being able to see that there is light despite all of the darkness.

Thank you for your time, Ray

I hope I get to hear this

Jonnie Kelly (Hopeful brother)

Ray turned to me. I explained that I had tried chemo and it hadn't worked, and I spoke about my quest to get access to Pembro. This was my last hope for survival, I told him.

Since putting up the page I had messages of support from all over the world. Somehow word had spread. There were people in Maryland offering me their homes to stay in if I went there, and offering me lifts to and from the hospital. People from all over Ireland had donated money and left messages of encouragement. The local community in Mooncoin had also organised a Midnight Walk, where the whole village turned out to walk by the light of the moon, in order to raise funds for my treatment. I thanked everyone who had written to me or donated or organised a fundraiser. It meant the world to me and my family, I told them.

Ray wound up the interview and thanked me for coming in. The text messages flooded in. People from around the country were offering their support. I was overwhelmed, I couldn't believe the response. I promised to stay in touch with the show, and to let them know how I was getting on.

People are just so good, I thought to myself, as Lyndsey and I made our way home. I suddenly felt less lonely, less isolated. There were people in my corner to help. I was energised by the experience.

The next day the researcher forwarded some of the emails that had come in to the station following the interview. I read through them, one by one. They were mainly from people who had been through cancer themselves, or had a loved one who had gone through treatment. They wanted to write to encourage me to keep going. I cried reading the emails. That human connection means so much when you're facing something like cancer. To know people were on my side, and that others had made it through, was such a comfort to me. It gave me strength and it spurred me on. It made me feel like I was doing the right thing.

I was reading through the messages when I stumbled upon an email that was a little bit different from the others. It was from a man named Peter. He hadn't heard the interview, but his mother-in-law had, and she had told him about it. He was getting in touch because his wife Emma was the exact same age as me and had died from cervical cancer just six weeks ago, he said. I took a deep breath. I wasn't sure if I was going to be able to read about someone who had died from the same cancer that I had, but I kept going. And thank God I did.

He went on to explain that Emma had wanted to try a different kind of treatment as well. She had looked into the trial in America that I was trying to get onto and had been accepted. Sadly, the treatment hadn't worked for her.

When I read that line, I fell apart. I was putting all my eggs in this basket, and some poor man who had just lost his wife was telling me that it hadn't worked.

The reason he was writing to me, he said, was because he wanted to help. He told me that while the trial didn't work for Emma, there were six other women on the trial and it had worked for four of them. He told me that he had all the contacts for the trial and that he would send me copies of Emma's files and talk me through the application she had sent in, and the trial itself, what it involved, etc. if I wanted to talk to someone about it.

In his email, Peter also told me that when his wife was no longer able to travel to America, she was offered Pembro on compassionate grounds, which was administered to her in Ireland. If I was interested, he said he would send me all the contact information and details about how Emma had received the drug, in order to help me to access something similar here while I was waiting to get on the trial.

My heart rate started to quicken. This was the best news I had received in a long time. If they had given one woman the drug on compassionate grounds, they should be able to do it again. It *was* possible to get Pembro for cervical cancer in Ireland. This piece of information was invaluable.

I wrote back to Peter immediately, thanking him for writing to me and for being so thoughtful, especially as he was still grieving the loss of his wife just six weeks ago. He told me that Emma would have wanted the information to help someone else. He was doing it for her.

Cancer audit process

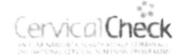

Case review

Name:	Ms Vicky Jane Phelan
Date of birth:	28 October 1974
Hospital ref	D316783

Identifier	CSP ID 1238520
Date of diagnosis:	15/07/2014
Review:	Cytology prior to diagnosis

Smear test date	Original report	Final review opinion
24/May/2011	NAD (no abnormality detected) Recommendation: Routine screening	Query squamous cell carcinoma

The original reporting laboratory participated in the cytology review and is aware of the outcomes. Please note that the final review opinion may follow review of the slide(s) by multiple laboratories whose opinions may differ.

Factors that should be borne in mind when considering these review outcomes include:

- the subjective nature of cytology interpretation
- the limitation of low sensitivity of cytology
- possible review bias ('hindsight bias' as the reason for review is known)
- reviews are not carried out under 'normal' screening conditions

The consultant pathologist for the original reporting laboratory should be consulted for each specific case.

The CervicalCheck audit report found on my file in January 2018, which set the wheels in motion for my subsequent court case and exposure of the CervicalCheck debacle.

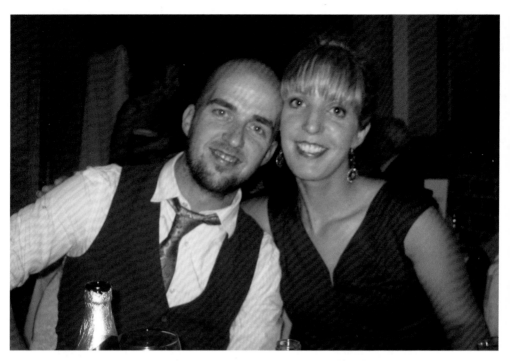

Me and my brother Jonnie in 2009. He emailed Ray D'Arcy's radio show about raising funds for me to take part in the NIH clinical trial in the US.

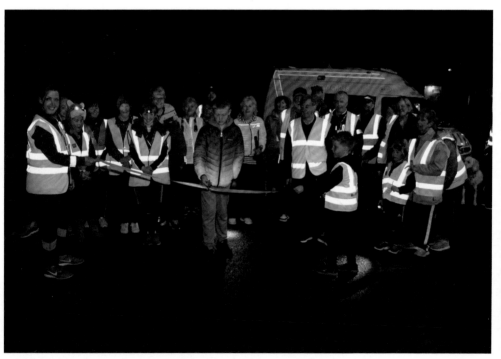

The Mooncoin Midnight Walk on 6 April 2018, which raised €24,000 for me to travel to the US.

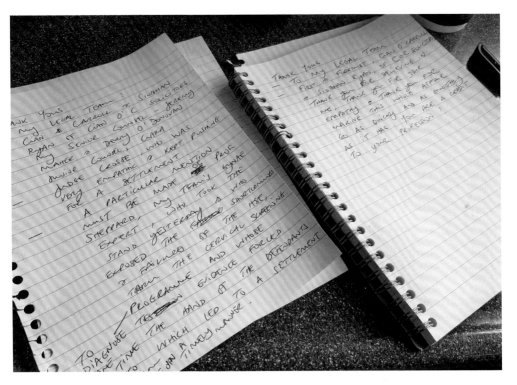

Writing my speech on the train to Dublin, on the morning of my settlement ruling, 25 April 2018.

Giving my statement to media at the Four Courts, Dublin.

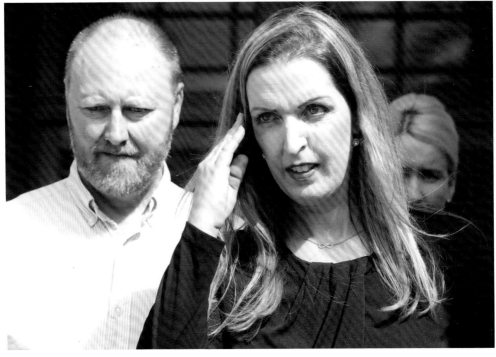

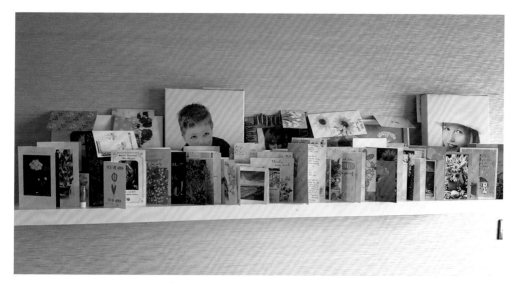

I've been so grateful to receive letters and cards of support from people all over the country since I went public on my case.

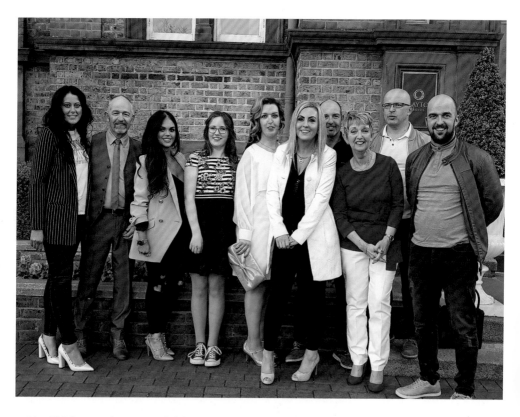

No TV interview would be complete without ... the entire family! Before my first TV appearance on The Ray D'Arcy Show, April 2018.

At the christening of my goddaughter Daisy Victoria, June 2019, a day I did not think I would be here to celebrate.

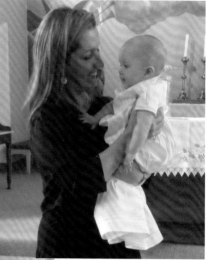

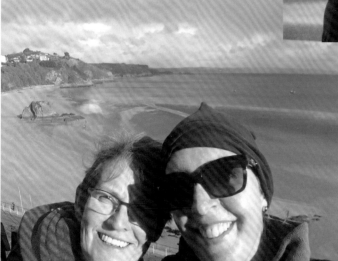

My good friend Eilish and I walking the Pembrokeshire Coastal Trail in Wales for our birthdays in October 2018. My friendships have kept me strong throughout my illness.

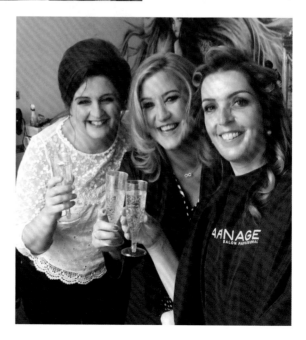

Myself and my best friends Susan, far left, and Maria, getting ready for a big night out.

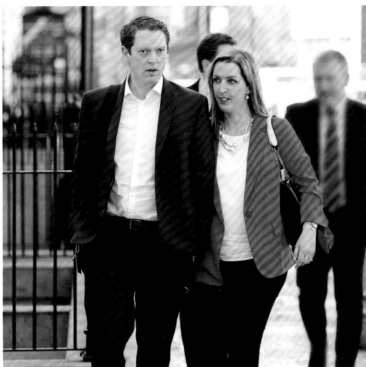

Stephen Teap and I on our way to Leinster House for our appearance at the Public Accounts Committee (PAC), 16 May 2018.

At the launch of the 221+ CervicalCheck Patient Support Group, with its founding members – Liz Yeates, Stephen McMahon, Lorraine Walsh, me, Stephen Teap, Donal Buggy, 14 October 2018.

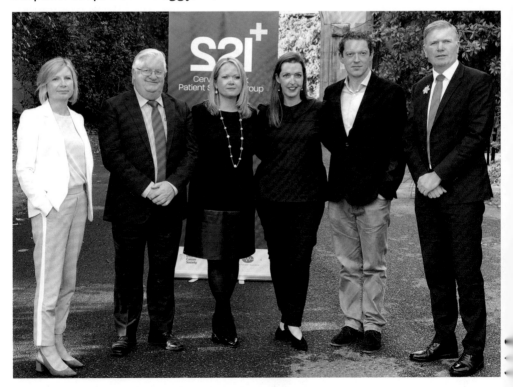

The first of many special days out – a private box was given to me and family and friends to enjoy the Munster v Edinburgh Pro14 match, 15 May 2018.

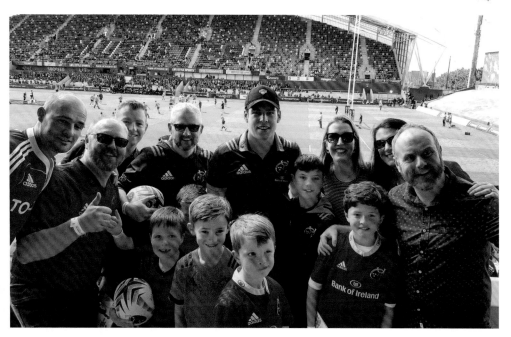

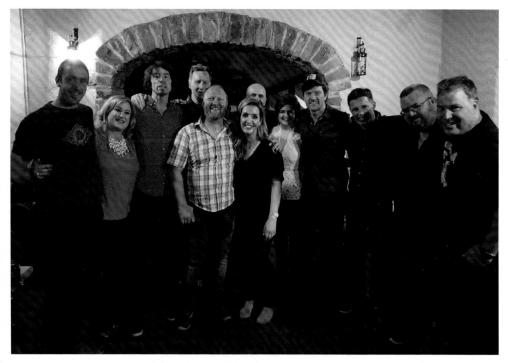

Me with some of my friends and The Stunning the night of our private gig in June 2018.

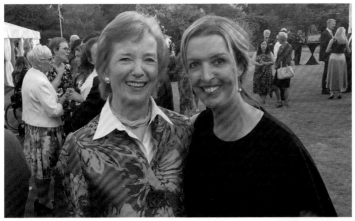

One of my heroes: meeting Mary Robinson at the British Ambassador's Summer Party, July 2018.

With Jim, my parents and Darragh on the day I received my Honorary Doctorate from University of Limerick, 26 June 2018.

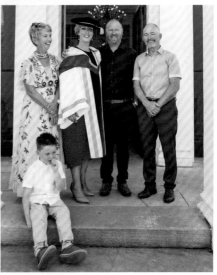

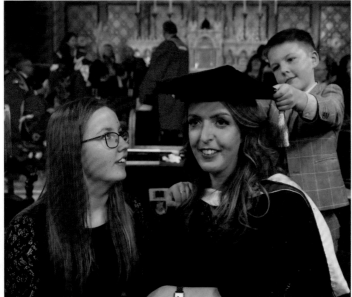

I was awarded an Honorary Fellowship by Waterford Institute of Technology in November 2018 and gave a speech on the importance of education. I hope my own children will appreciate its importance as they grow up.

It felt like I had been given a lifeline all of a sudden – a glimmer of hope as the clock counted down. I remembered the oncologist's words: six months without chemotherapy. I was on borrowed time.

33

Zipped Lips

T HE PHONE RANG. IT WAS Cian.
      'Vicky, can you sit down somewhere?'
'What's happened?'
'We've just got the files back from CervicalCheck. There are fourteen other women, Vicky. Siobhan and I have been sitting here, wondering how we were going to tell you this. Your name was on this spreadsheet, so anything you were mentioned in, legally, had to be sent to us. They had blacked out the other names.' He explained that the patients were listed from 'A' to 'O'. I was 'Patient M'.

The report I had found in my file in the hospital was also included. It was sent from the head of CervicalCheck, to my doctor. The missing page 1 revealed that it had been sent in July 2016, fourteen months before I was told anything about the audit. When my solicitors looked at the correspondence it showed that there were fourteen women in total. And my doctor had only been instructed that there were three women that he could tell. I thought back to the moment the doctor had told me about the audit. I suddenly felt thankful to him for informing me. He had gone against the advice of CervicalCheck and decided to tell all of his patients.

If the women were dead, the consultants were instructed to simply put a note on their file. I wondered if that meant there were families around the country, missing a mum or a wife who had died, who might never know that the death of their loved one could have been prevented.

There were other women involved, and we now had proof.

I felt determined that this needed to be brought to public attention. These women and their families had a right to know the truth.

We had been invited by the defendants to come to a mediation hearing, which was set for 9 April. At that point, Cian said he would bet his house we wouldn't go to court. He was sure we would settle at the hearing.

I always imagined mediation would involve people sitting around a long table, 'clients' represented by solicitors putting forward their offers and proffers and counter-offers. I think my idea of it came from all those American movies where you see the couples going through divorce proceedings, awkwardly sitting opposite one another, dividing assets and settling custody arrangements. So when Jim and I arrived at the Distillery Building in Dublin, where mediation hearings take place, I was very surprised by the set-up. It would almost have been comical, only that it was so serious.

Cian met us in the lobby and brought us to the cafeteria for a coffee. He told us that they weren't quite ready for us yet but that he would come down and fetch us when it was time to get started. He explained that there were three rooms, with each party in a room of their own – me, the HSE and the lab the smear had been sent to for testing – each with their respective teams of lawyers around them. A mediator would go from one room to the next to put offers on the table, and relay the replies. None of us would see each other throughout the encounter.

He also told us that we would be meeting our senior and junior counsel. When you take a court case and it goes to trial, your solicitor has to engage the services of barristers, who argue the case for the plaintiff. I would have two senior counsel, Jeremy Maher and Derry O'Donovan, arguing my case, since there were two defendants. The more people you are suing, the more barristers you need. There would also be a junior counsel, Ciara McGoldrick, who would assist the senior counsel with preparing for the case. Today would give Jim and me an opportunity to be briefed by Jeremy and Derry on what to expect from the trial, if it went to court. Our hope was that it would settle that day, and we wouldn't need to go any further.

It was the barristers' job to negotiate at mediation hearings. The glass was frosted so that you couldn't see into the next room. I took a seat and tried to get comfortable. I was in a lot of pain and had taken strong painkillers to try to make it through the day. I had my hot-water bottle on the seat behind my back. I still wasn't on any medication and I had been feeling very sick as the cancer quietly crept through my body. While we waited, Jeremy and Derry talked us through giving evidence and began asking me questions, as I would be the first one to take the stand, should my case go to court.

We waited for word to come from one of the other rooms. Finally, there was a knock on the door. The mediator arrived.

He said he wanted to bring all parties around the table to discuss the options. Cian was adamant this was not going to happen. It would be very unusual for a plaintiff in such a sensitive medical negligence case to have to sit opposite the defendants. With that, the mediator left. We waited to see what would happen next. A few minutes later, he came back into the room with the mediation agreement which had been sent to my lawyers earlier in the week. I was told that it was common practice to agree that anything that was discussed in mediation was confidential and couldn't be used in court if the mediation was unsuccessful. Normally this is signed on the day. However, there was something very different about this agreement. The other parties were seeking an amendment with a new clause that required that I agree to absolute confidentiality of any settlement.

'They want you to sign a confidentiality clause,' Cian said.

'What does that mean, exactly?' I asked.

'They won't discuss any deal or settlement unless you sign to say that you will not tell anyone anything about this.'

I thought about that dotted line that I would have to sign. Like an ellipsis ... the ellipsis of the story of my life. To be continued ...

But that's just the thing, I thought. My life won't be continued. This might be the full stop, where the story ends, because of what happened to me. The irony of that ellipsis made me angry. And what about the other women, or the families of those who may already have died. The lives that had already come to an end. If I signed, they would never know the truth.

'I can't sign that,' I said to Cian.

He looked at me for a moment

'I won't do it.' I was adamant.

'Then we go public,' he said. 'But you need to be prepared for what that means.'

I looked at him to explain.

'It means going to court. It means talking about a lot of personal things, in front of court reporters.'

'People need to know,' I said, eventually.

'And your health?'

'I have to do this, for my sanity.'

But would I be *able* to do it, that was the question on everyone's minds, though no one said it.

Cian asked me, straight, 'What do you want out of this?'

'First of all, I want an apology. I would also like someone to admit that they made a mistake, but I don't think I'll get that.'

'An admission of liability? No, I don't think you will.'

'And beyond that, I just want enough money to cover my family if I don't survive this.'

'This could get nasty,' he said.

I tried to brace myself. I took a deep breath. The lawyers looked at me for an answer.

'No.'

'Are you sure, Vicky?' Cian said.

'Certain.'

Cian relayed the decision to the mediator, who was then charged with going to the next room to tell the other parties.

I was happy that we had stuck to our guns. Now it was game on. We had shown them we weren't in it for the money. This was about a lot more than that. If they thought we could be bought off, they had another thing coming.

There was a knock on the door. The mediator was back.

We all turned to look at him.

He gave us the return message from the other parties: no

chance of a settlement if the non-disclosure agreement was not signed.

I shook my head. I was standing firm.

This went on for hours. I maintained my position. The day felt long.

It was like a game of poker – waiting to see who would fold first.

Finally, the day came to a close. No offer was forthcoming, and I steadfastly refused to sign. Stalemate.

Cian looked anxious.

'I suppose this means we're going to court?' I said.

'I'm afraid so.'

Jim and I drove home to Limerick. I was tired after a long day. It was hard to concentrate on anything. I got into bed with my hot-water bottle and closed my eyes.

The following morning, I heard the familiar 'ding' of an email in my inbox. Bleary eyed, I checked my phone. It was from NIH in Maryland. I sat up. They were writing to inform me that the results had come back from my blood test and unfortunately, even though I ticked all the other boxes, I didn't have this one particular type of protein in my blood. I was not eligible for the clinical trial.

I read the email aloud to Jim. His legs nearly went from under him. He lay across the bed, with his head in my lap. 'What are we going to do now, Vicky?'

I didn't have an answer. I was crying uncontrollably. We were both broken from the weight of the news. We were now facing into a legal trial we had hoped would not come to pass, and I had been rejected from the clinical trial I had so desperately wanted.

I was running out of options. I tried to gather myself, and get back on my laptop. It was the only thing I could think of to do. I searched and searched and found another clinical trial – in Buffalo, New York. It was a similar trial, but this one was even more expensive. I began the application process again, hoping this time I might get a different result.

34

Judgement Day

IT WAS NOW THREE MONTHS since I was told that I only had six months to live without treatment. Their predictions seemed to be accurate. The pain was unbearable and my stomach was getting bigger by the day. I was wearing maternity clothes to fit my swollen belly as my 10-centimetre tumour was bulging through my abdomen.

Somehow I had to believe there was a solution. It wasn't denial, so much as a coping mechanism. But I was starting to lose hope. Thoughts of death were going through my head. I was too young to die. My children were too young to lose their mother. But there was no masking the reality. I was feeling sick. Very sick. I could feel the cancer taking over, slowly getting the better of me.

It was the Friday before the court case. I was trying to prepare myself, mentally, for what the next week had in store. I was sitting in the recliner when I received a phone call. Dr

Fennelly's number. I was almost too tired to pick up the phone, but I answered, hesitantly.

'Hello?'

'Good news, Vicky,' said Dr Fennelly.

At last, I thought. I held my breath.

He told me the hospital had finally approved my prescription for Pembro. I would be getting my first infusion the following Monday, 16 April, three days before I was due to give evidence in court. I was nearly too sick to feel relieved; I was exhausted. I thanked him and hung up and fell asleep again.

That Sunday, 15 April, was my father's birthday. I really wanted to make it down to Kilkenny to celebrate it with him and the rest of the family. We planned to leave Amelia and Darragh with Mam and Dad after the birthday lunch. Then we would drive to Dublin and stay overnight at a hotel near St Vincent's Hospital, as I had to be there early on Monday morning to have bloods taken before my infusion.

I never fully understood how sick I really was until that day. I fell asleep in the passenger seat of the car on the journey down. I was drifting in and out of a deep sleep the whole way. I felt disorientated.

We arrived at Jack Meade's pub for the lunch. I got out of the car and walked slowly across the car park, leaning on Jim's arm for support. The whole family were sitting at a table under the awning outside: Mam and Dad, and my sister and brothers and their partners and children. They turned to look at me. I'll never forget the terrified look on their faces as they saw me walking towards them.

'Do I look that bad?' I asked Jim, quietly.

He couldn't bring himself to lie. 'Not great, Vicky ...' he said, rubbing my arm. That almost broke me.

Seeing the look on my family's faces, I wondered if I had done the right thing. Had I played Russian roulette with my life? Had I left it too late to get on Pembro? Were the doctors' predictions going to come true? Would I make it to the end of my court case? All these questions were racing through my mind.

We reached the table and Mam made room for me to sit beside her, propping a cushion up behind me. I barely lasted until the main course was served. Mam turned to me. 'You're not comfortable there, Vicky, are you?' She could see I was in pain.

'No ...' I said. I was trying to be brave, for Dad, for his birthday, but I was in agony.

I gave Dad a hug and Mam brought me home to lie down. I was uncomfortable and I was exhausted.

After I had rested at my parents' house, Jim came into the room. 'Are you sure you're okay to go to Dublin?' he asked.

I could barely sit up in the bed. 'Yes,' I said. After everything I had gone through to get access to the drug, I couldn't bear the thought of missing the appointment.

Jim helped me out to the car and we travelled to Dublin later that evening. We checked into the hotel, and I slept through the night. The next morning, I woke early. I got dressed and caught sight of my reflection in the long hotel mirror. It was the first time I had stopped to look at myself in a long time. I could see what they saw. My eyes had black rings underneath them. I was pale and weak and my tumours were pushing my stomach out so much, I looked like I was eight months pregnant.

I splashed some water on my face and walked out the door. When we arrived at the hospital car park, Jim said, 'Wait here, I'll get a wheelchair.'

'No, I'll walk,' I said stubbornly. I needed to walk in there myself, on my own two feet. I needed to believe that I was not dying.

It was a long morning waiting for the results of my bloods to come back before the nurses gave the go-ahead for my Pembro to be ordered from the lab. When the medication arrived, I couldn't believe how small the pouch was. I looked at it – this liquid I had fought so hard to get. The pouch had just 200 ml of fluid in it. How could this little bag of liquid cost 8,500 euro per dose, I wondered. I closed my eyes while the nurse injected it into my arm. I imagined the medicine coursing through my veins. This wonder drug I had prayed for, finally finding its way into my body. I wondered if it was too late. Or if I still stood a chance of survival.

Later that night, after we got home to Limerick, my temperature spiked. I seemed to be having an adverse reaction to the drug. No, I thought to myself, this can't be happening. This is the drug that is supposed to save me.

I began hallucinating. Jim stayed by my side. We were both afraid. We'd never experienced anything like this before. I was drifting in and out of consciousness. I have very little memory of what happened that night. It was a night of hell. Jim monitored my temperature and fed me paracetamol at regular intervals.

The worst seemed to be over by 6 a.m. I started to come round. I was conscious again, but I felt sick to my core. I was vomiting and had a severe headache and aches and pains everywhere, as if I had the worst flu of my life. At 8 a.m., as soon as the ward opened at St Vincent's, Jim got on the phone and spoke to a nurse to explain what had happened. I was aware that Jim was on the phone. I could hear him, but it felt like I was somewhere else. The nurse explained to Jim that some patients can experience a severe reaction to Pembro.

It was now Tuesday. The trial was starting on Thursday. I couldn't function. How could I possibly sit in court and give evidence? I had hoped the opposite would be true – that the Pembro would have given me a burst of energy, to get through the next few days.

Siobhan, our solicitor, called Jim to see how I was doing. I could hear him telling her that there was no way I'd be able to go to Dublin on Thursday. Cian and Siobhan had held out hope that the case would still settle out of court. No settlement came, and with two days to go, the trial was definitely going ahead. I asked Jim to pass me the phone.

'I don't think I will be able to make it …' I told Siobhan from my recliner.

At that point I could barely stand up, let alone make a trip to Dublin.

Siobhan reassured me that my health had to come first.

They were trying not to pressurise me, but we all knew there was a lot at stake if I couldn't make it.

I tried to make my peace with not being at the trial. If I wasn't able to go, then I just couldn't be there. Simple as that. It was out of my control. But I was restless at the thought. We had come so far. We had put so much work into this. I hated to think of the case defeating me, of the cancer getting one over on us. I had fought so hard for the chance to tell my story, and now I felt like I was being silenced by the disease.

Wednesday, 18 April, the day before the trial. I woke in a sweat. I was so weak, but I couldn't bear the thought of letting it all slip away. If I died without seeing this case go to court, I would die without answers – answers for me and all the other women affected.

While Jim was out collecting the kids from school, I picked up the phone and rang Cian and Siobhan.

'I'm not sure how,' I said, 'but I'm going to make it to court tomorrow to tell my side of the story. If it's the last thing I do …'

That evening, Jim and I made our way to Dublin. We left Amelia and Darragh in the care of our neighbours and friends, who were all rooting for us and supporting us all the way. Cian had booked a hotel room for us around the corner from the courthouse. When we arrived I closed the curtains and got into bed, under the duvet with my hot-water bottle. I was in and out of sleep all night. The nerves, on top of feeling ill, were making it impossible to switch off. Every time I woke, I looked at the time: 2 a.m. … then 3 a.m. … 4.30 a.m.

Light began to stream through the gap in the curtains. It was Thursday, 19 April, the day of the trial. I pulled the duvet over my head. I felt like screaming into the pillow. I had always imagined I would be strong the day we came to court. I had played it out in my mind a hundred times. Now, I wasn't sure how I was going to get through the day, let alone give my testimony.

It took all of my strength to get dressed and to put on my makeup, to take that yellow sick-person look off my face, the look that I could now see, staring back at me in the mirror.

The moment had finally arrived. We walked out of the hotel and made our way slowly to the Four Courts. The river Liffey looked beautiful that day as we walked alongside it; the light was shimmering off it. The water was comforting. It was calm in the midst of the bustling traffic and my racing mind.

Jim and I arrived at the courthouse. I could see that my

parents and Maria and Susan and my aunts Ann and Kathleen and Uncle Frankie were already there, nervously waiting.

Jim gave me a hug. 'Good luck,' he said.

'Thank you,' I replied. And I meant it. No one really knew, except us, what we had been through – in the middle of the night when temperatures were spiking, and when bad news was coming in by email. Only we knew all of that. He held me for a moment, then turned and followed my family and friends to be seated in the gallery.

I checked myself and took a deep breath. Cian and Siobhan walked over to me. We hugged. 'Good luck, Vicky. We're behind you all the way,' they said. And I knew that they were.

I walked through the heavy double doors of the courtroom and all eyes turned towards me. I could feel the room watching me. They must have been surprised to see me there. I felt a surge of energy all of a sudden. I was ready for them. If they thought they could push me until I'd back down, or that I'd be too sick to fight, they didn't know who they were dealing with.

When it was my turn to take the stand, I was nervous. I had never set foot in a courtroom before. It was all very different to how I had imagined it. I slowly walked up to where the plaintiff sits. The wooden seat was hard and uncomfortable. I placed my hot-water bottle behind me, lodged against my back. I tried to look strong, but I was grimacing with the pain.

I was seated at a height, directly opposite the stenographer, who would record everything I said. I looked down at the courtroom. Cian and Siobhan were there, but I could only see the backs of their heads. The court was set up so that your lawyers are turned away from you when you are on the stand. I wasn't expecting this. It threw me. They were the people I trusted and needed for reassurance. I was on my own now.

It was all about hierarchy in the courtroom. The judge was at a height at the top of the room. I was below him, to the side, and then all the lawyers were below that again seated at a long table.

Judge Cross was very compassionate, making it clear that proceedings could be stalled whenever I needed a break.

Jeremy Maher, one of my senior counsel, opened by summing up my life to the court. It was strange to sit there and listen to it all – the story of my life: Victoria Kelly was born in Waterford on 28 October 1974. Back to where it all began. They told the court about my education, at national and secondary school and then on to university, where I received a first-class honours degree. My studies were interrupted for a period, they told the court, by a car accident in France in 1994, in which two other passengers died, and in which I sustained various injuries.

I thought of Christophe, and of Lisa.

I recovered from this, they told the court, and later went on to complete a master's degree. I had married a man named Jim, the other plaintiff in this case. He was a carpenter who worked mainly with his father. He had recently completed a degree. They talked about the birth of my daughter Amelia, and about her condition, and about the fire. Then came my son Darragh, born several years later. They talked about work – where I had worked and what positions I had had. All the things that had happened, to bring me to the day I had my smear test in 2011, and the letter I had received to tell me that the smear was normal. This is where this story began.

The questioning was gruelling. I took two breaks in the morning and one in the afternoon.

What happens is, you are asked questions by your barristers and then the other side can cross-examine. I was anxious about the cross-examining – that's the big unknown. Though there was a lot that couldn't be disputed – they couldn't dispute that I had cancer that could have been cured in 2011, but which was now terminal. But regardless of those cold, hard facts, things could get very messy and personal.

The cross-examining began. I've heard it described as being like a dance, where everyone knows the next step, but you. And that's exactly how it felt.

My lawyers had warned me to expect the worst. They said it would all boil down to my loss of earnings. And it did. It came down to money. Not life, or the value of it. How can anyone put a value on life? It was all about trying to weigh up my worth. It was sickening.

I was exhausted. The judge proposed that we could recess and come back the following day if I was finding it too difficult. I appreciated that. He was very understanding. But no, I wasn't coming back. It had to be now. I needed to get this done, once and for all.

A barrister for the lab started asking me questions about work.

I began talking through my day. Initially, it didn't occur to me where he was going with this.

Then when he asked about what happened each week when I went to Waterford for work, I started to explain what my average week looked like. I told him that I worked from home two days a week and in Waterford for the other three days. I explained that I travelled to Waterford on a Monday morning, stayed Monday and Tuesday, and came back to Limerick on Wednesday evening, and that when in Waterford I usually stayed with my parents or with my sister, as they lived close to my workplace.

He quickly replied, questioning what childcare arrangements I had in place, as Jim had recently started working again. I explained that we had a lady who came to the house in the morning, made the kids' breakfast and brought them to school. Then when school was over, they went to an after-school club and my husband picked them up from there and brought them home. That was our usual routine.

Then he asked how the kids were getting on with this arrangement. He talked about their hobbies – Amelia liked swimming, and reading, and writing. He asked if they were socialising well.

To which I answered, yes.

And then it suddenly dawned on me what he was doing. Or at least, what I thought he was doing. I'll never know for sure. Was he trying to imply that if I died, the children would be okay? That there'd be somebody there to mind them?

Cian had warned me that it was all going to become very personal. And that's what was happening. My face went red with anger. My parents could see that something had aggravated me. They could see the veins on my neck pulsating.

I can't say it was intended that way, but running through my mind in the moment was, how could anyone think that my childminder could possibly replace me? My childminder did not carry Amelia and Darragh for nine months, or go through two years of hardship when Amelia was born, giving her carefully weighed-out medication three times a day, taking her to occupational therapy, speech and language therapy and appointments with infectious diseases consultants and ophthalmologists. My childminder was not the one who slept beside Darragh most nights when he was little and afraid, or who knew the bedtime stories that he liked to send him to sleep.

I was furious. I wasn't sure how much of this I could take. It was exhausting.

Finally the proceedings were called to a close and I went straight back to the hotel. As I lay in bed, I replayed every question in my head. I tried to remember how I had answered them. I thought about it until I drifted off to sleep.

We went home to Limerick that evening as we had a big occasion ahead of us the next day. It was Amelia's confirmation, an important day in her life and one that we were looking forward to celebrating with our families. I stayed in Limerick for the remainder of the trial. I was back in my recliner, resting. Cian and Siobhan kept me updated every day by phone so that I knew how things were progressing.

Jim was due to take the stand on Tuesday. The thought of it was terrifying him. We were both at home the day before. I heard a noise – it was Jim struggling to breathe. He was having a panic attack. I tried to calm him down, and then he started again. He was having an attack every few minutes, where he was short of breath.

I rang the GP. 'He's going up to give evidence in court tomorrow. He's in an awful state. I'm afraid he's going to have a heart attack or something. Can you give him something to calm him down?' I asked.

He was prescribed Xanax to calm his nerves. I watched him pacing around the house all afternoon. I felt guilty for putting him through this.

We decided it would be best if I stayed in Limerick. If I was in the courtroom he would feel even more nervous; it'd be easier for him if I wasn't there, if I wasn't listening. We were anticipating questions about our personal life, our relationship and our sex life. Jim is a very private person. The thought of going through all those emotions in front of a court full of strangers, with aggressive questioning from lawyers, would be enough to make anyone feel sick.

'You need to have someone with you, though, Jim. You can't go by yourself,' I said, handing him a glass of water.

I rang his good friend Dara. I knew he would relax Jim and put him at ease. I asked if he would accompany him to court. He was very supportive and assured me he would do anything he could to help.

On Tuesday morning, Dara arrived at the house to collect Jim for the journey.

I stopped Jim as he was walking out the door. 'Thank you for doing this.' I gave him a hug.

I stood in the doorway and watched as he got into the car. I couldn't believe this was really happening to us. How dare they make my husband get up on the stand to talk about his wife dying and the effect it has had on our marriage, and on our family, and how he's going to be able to cope without her. It was the worst part of it all. I knew he would do anything for me – he was even prepared to do this.

I waved them off and mouthed the words 'thank you'. I knew Jim was in safe hands with Dara. He would keep him distracted on the train ride to Dublin and would be a great support for Jim.

I went to the kitchen to make a cup of coffee. I tried to imagine the kinds of things they might ask. It made me feel angry to think of Jim up on the stand, feeling vulnerable while strangers asked him intimate questions about our personal life. He didn't deserve this. It was bad enough that I had to do it. The thoughts of one of my family having to do it as well infuriated me. Jim would be first to take the stand that day. I set myself up in the recliner chair and placed the phone beside me. I wanted to be on call in case he needed to talk to me.

Jim and Dara arrived at the Four Courts. Jim was shaking and finding it difficult to talk; he was trying hard to hold it together. Dara was doing his best to calm his nerves. Jim took some more Xanax.

One of the lawyers was coming towards him as he sat on the courthouse bench. He took a deep breath and braced himself, assuming they were coming to ask him to take the stand. Instead, they asked if he would mind waiting until later to give his testimony. Jim breathed a sigh of relief. That would be fine, he told them.

Then official word came from the judge, to say that there would be a change in the order of the day. Professor John Shepherd was a retired consultant gynaecological oncologist and was one of our expert witnesses. He had reviewed the case history and written a report on the matter. He would take the stand first. He had flown in from Wales for the trial. He was scheduled to appear after Jim, but he needed to catch a flight back home in the evening so they had requested that he go first. Jim gladly obliged.

The court had heard from my lawyers, who claimed that the alleged failure to diagnose the 2011 smear test sample caused a situation whereby my cancer went unidentified, unmonitored and untreated, developing and spreading, until I was diagnosed with the disease in July 2014. My cancer went from one that could have been cured, to one that was terminal.

Professor Shepherd was called as a witness. His testimony was powerful.

'If the smear had been correctly reported in 2011, the cancer would not have developed?' he was asked.

'On the balance of probability, that is correct,' he replied.

'And had the smear been correctly reported in 2011, Ms Phelan would have a normal life expectancy?'

'She would have had a normal life expectancy taking into account her overall medical state, yes.'

He confirmed that I would not have had to undergo chemotherapy, brachytherapy or radiotherapy and that there was a high probability that I would have been cured. In relation to my smear test, he said it was 'one of a number of smears that had been reviewed and found to be wanting'.

On the issue of how the findings of the audit were not communicated to me, various letters between my doctor and CervicalCheck were read out, including one from my doctor to the head of CervicalCheck dated 28 July 2016:

... As part of Cervical Cancer Audit, we were asked to review notes for ladies who subsequently were diagnosed with either invasive cancer or in situ carcinoma. This was in light of a review of the cytology showing a difference on the original report. We have reviewed all these notes and are happy that their clinical management since attending us in the colposcopy unit has been appropriate and all ladies are thankfully alive and well and undergoing follow-up. We feel it inappropriate for us to contact them at this point to tell them their original smears have been re-reported as showing different findings and we think that this would only heighten their anxiety levels and not confer any advantage to them now in their clinical course as they have all been managed appropriately. However, I

think it is the responsibility for CervicalCheck to judge for themselves as to whether they have responsibility to these ladies to call them and acknowledge the alteration in their original smears after review.

When asked if he had a view on the opinion expressed by the doctor, Professor Shepherd said, '... I would have to disagree with his decision and that of presumably the colleagues that he has discussed this with. They have been given the responsibility of advising and treating a number of patients, a number of ladies, and I think that it's their responsibility to correctly inform them of any errors that have occurred, even if they believe that these individual ladies have not come to any harm.'

There was a reply to the doctor on 5 August 2016 written by the National Screening Service:

It's good to hear that these women are doing well. Etc In the information for healthcare professionals, we recognise that there is a balance in terms of communicating the result of an audit, particularly where women are unaware of its existence. This balance is best judged by the clinician who knows the patients and who has been looking after the woman, taking into consideration the individual clinical context. It is therefore up to you as clinical lead to use your clinical judgment with regard to these individual reports.

Then they read from various letters that followed, including a letter from my doctor to the head of CervicalCheck, dated 22 August 2017, over a year later.

I strongly believe that CervicalCheck, who conducted this whole audit process, should have communicated directly to the women involved, detailing that their smear test prior to their diagnoses of cervical cancer had been reviewed and showed a significant altered finding which could have impacted on their ultimate treatment.

... It is because I feel that the women deserve to know the results of the audit process, I have taken it upon myself to go through the results of the audit with them as they return for their follow-up clinic visits.

It seemed he had pushed the programme to disclose the information to us for over a year, then made the decision to tell us himself.

The letters were read and put to Professor Shepherd for his opinion. Of the delay in the information about the audit being communicated to me, he said that, in his opinion, it seemed 'most irregular' and absolutely should not happen.

In his examination of the records he could see that a review was undertaken by the CervicalCheck screening programme in 2014 which uncovered the false negative result, but that this was not communicated to me, the patient, until 2017. 'I think that there is a moral and ethical responsibility on all professionals (and in this case the doctors and clinicians involved) to notify the patient of any errors that have occurred,' he said.

Lawyers for the HSE made the point that one of the reasons for the delay in my being informed was because they were completing a review which went back to 2008, hence it took some time to deal with those affected by 2011 tests.

The court was told that CervicalCheck informed my doctors

about the mistake in 2016 but that there was a further delay until 2017 before I was told.

In relation to the documents about the audit, Professor Shepherd said they seemed 'confusing' and there was no direct guidance as to how the situation should be dealt with.

He was asked about correspondence between CervicalCheck and my doctors, and those of other women. From the communication between CervicalCheck and my doctors, there seemed to be a difference of opinion about who should inform me and other patients of the mistakes that had been uncovered. Professor Shepherd said that, in his opinion, by telling doctors to use their clinical judgment, the screening service was 'ducking the issue'. He also agreed during cross-examination that there was no malice or lack of bona fides involved in the process.

It was put to him that the only person who did not seem to have been involved in this correspondence was me. Professor Shepherd agreed and said that I had been 'totally ignored' and that that should not have happened.

What was his opinion, he was asked, on the fact that no one seemed to be taking responsibility for telling me about the original mistake.

In his expert opinion, he said, he felt that this was 'unacceptable' and that an overarching body should have been set up by the HSE to advise on this.

The atmosphere was suddenly very different in the courtroom.

All of this was happening unbeknownst to me. I was sitting in my recliner at home, nervously waiting for news, when my phone rang. It was Cian.

'Is everything okay?' I asked. 'How is Jim getting on?'

'They want to settle, Vicky,' he said.

I couldn't believe it. The case was over. He told me that Professor Shepherd had blown them all out of the water. Cian said they were practically running for cover.

They were offering to settle, for a sum of 2.5 million euro, but without an admission of liability.

I had secured a huge victory by my determination to fight the defendants until the precondition of confidentiality was removed. This paved the way for other women and families to take cases and to expose the failings of the CervicalCheck screening programme. And for that, I was so very grateful.

I wondered if we should push harder, to see if we could get an admission of liability. But then we agreed: this was where we drew the line. The case was over. The job was done.

35

Victim Impact

THE FOLLOWING MORNING I TRAVELLED to Dublin to attend the final day in court, to rule the settlement.

The night before, Cian and I had spoken about making a statement to the media. I assumed that this was something that Cian would do, as my solicitor. Cian felt, however, that the media would want to hear from me and that the women of Ireland would want to hear from me. I had an important message and I was the best person to deliver that message. I asked him what I should say. He asked me how I felt. I told him that I felt angry, and that I had lost all trust in our screening programme.

I wrote my speech on the train to Dublin that morning, scribbled on one of my daughter's notepads. I wrote from the heart. I poured my feelings onto the page and then I went back over what I had written to make sense of it.

When we were back in the courtroom, Judge Kevin Cross said that he was delighted that the case was officially settled. I could return to normal life with my family now and concentrate on fighting my cancer. He turned to me and said, 'If anyone can beat this, you can.' I smiled and thanked him.

It was finally over. Cian and Siobhan ushered Jim and me into a consultation room to prepare us for the media scrum that was waiting for us outside. I ran my statement by Cian, who said that it was perfect.

'Ready?' he asked.

'I'm ready,' I said.

We all hugged. It was an emotional moment for all four of us, who had been through so much together over the past ten weeks.

I walked out onto the steps of the courthouse. There was a crowd of people gathered. I could hear the clicking of cameras coming from every direction as journalists huddled around me.

Cian pointed me towards the plinth. The reporters held out microphones in front of me. I could feel Jim's hand on the small of my back as he stood beside me, a reminder of his constant support. I took a breath. I felt exhausted. I took out the statement I had prepared and read it aloud.

To my family and friends and my supporters who supported my decision to take this case at a time I really should be concentrating on my health, I would not have been able to do this without you.

There are no winners here today. I am terminally ill and there is no cure for my cancer. My settlement will mostly be spent on buying me time and on paying for clinical trials to keep me alive and to allow me spend more time with my children.

I was trying hard not to cry, but the emotion of the day was building up inside me.

If I die – and I truly hope that won't be the case – the money will provide for my family.

The women of Ireland can no longer put their trust in the CervicalCheck programme. Mistakes can and do happen, but the conduct of CervicalCheck and the HSE in my case, and in the case of at least ten other women that we know about, is unforgiveable. To know for almost three years that a mistake had been made and that I was misdiagnosed was bad enough, but to keep that information from me until I became terminally ill and to drag me through the courts for my right to the truth is an appalling breach of trust.

I truly hope that some good will come of this case and that there will be an investigation into the CervicalCheck programme as a result of this.

I thanked my lawyers for all their hard work. I felt so grateful to Cian and Siobhan for being by my side through it all. It was because of them that the world would know what had happened, to ensure that it could never happen again.

We wanted to escape the furore of the press. I was still feeling very weak, so we left and went to the Marker Hotel in Grand Canal Square. The Marker, I thought, looking at the embossed logo on the room service menu. It was ironic. In cancer, you live and die by your 'markers' – always hoping the markers in your blood are doing well. Perhaps it is a good luck sign, I thought.

That night I slept soundly, for the first time in a long time.

The next morning I saw *The Irish Times* in the lobby, with my photograph on the front page. This is big, I thought to myself. Until now, it had been something between me and my lawyers and the HSE. Now it suddenly felt different. My phone was buzzing. The texts had been flooding in all morning. News was spreading.

I read the report. 'Mr Justice Kevin Cross has described Ms Phelan as the most impressive witness he had ever encountered.' I couldn't believe what I was reading. I'm sure he has seen a lot of things in his time, I thought. I felt a surge of appreciation for this man, whose role was to find the truth, to allow justice to prevail.

The report continued:

He also praised both sides in the case for the speed with which the case was handled. In her High Court action, which began last week, her lawyers said if the cancerous cells had been detected in 2011 she would have had a simple procedure and would have a 90% chance of survival.

Ms Phelan, of Carrigeen, Annacotty, Co. Limerick along with her husband Jim Phelan has sued the Health Service Executive and Clinical Pathology Laboratories Inc, Austin, Texas, over a smear test taken under the National Screening Programme CervicalCheck and analysed in the US laboratory.

The court was told the case had now settled and the case against the HSE could be struck out with no order.

The settlement with the US laboratory for €2.5 million was made without admission of liability. A portion of the settlement will be paid into court and be held for the couple's two children who are now aged seven and 12.

It was surreal reading about my family in the news, seeing our names, our address – our home there for all to read. It was all there in black and white, but it felt as though they were talking about someone else. Someone else's family, someone else's life.

I put down the paper. I felt like I could breathe for the first time in a long time. The truth was known. I just hoped some good would come of this for the women of Ireland.

36

The Promise

THE FOLLOWING EVENING WE WERE back in our own home – the four of us. I went upstairs to tuck the children into bed and say goodnight. I found Amelia sitting on her bed, crying.

'What's wrong, petto?' I put my arm around her.

I could almost hear the thoughts and worries building up in her head. She sniffled, and eventually, catching her breath through tears, she said, 'Mam ...'

'Yes, petto.'

'Are you going to die, Mammy?'

'I don't know, Amelia.' I closed my eyes and pulled her closer to me. 'There's a chance that I could die.' I needed to be honest with her. I've always been honest with her.

I knew she was seeing the news headlines. I was being referred to in the media as a 'terminally ill woman' and 'dying' and 'sentenced to death' and she was picking up on it all.

'But you know your mammy, I'm a fighter. Like you, Amelia.

We'll get there, petto. This is what the money is for, for me to go off on all these clinical trials. I'll be here for as long as I can. I promise you that.'

I waited until she was asleep, kissed her goodnight and went downstairs. The kitchen light was out. I left it off. There was something calming about being in the quiet of the darkness. I made a cup of tea and sat at the kitchen table. It is the hardest part of it all, the kids. It goes against all my instincts to see them upset. Darragh is only a baby. He's just seven, but he picks up on everything too.

I looked at the card he had made for me that week. 'I'm wrd about you Mammy,' it said. 'When is your belly going to be better?' He knows I have cancer in my belly.

'I promise I'll be here as long as I can. I promise you that,' I whispered in the darkness. I needed to do everything in my power to keep that promise.

37

The Others

I HAD SOME SOLACE IN knowing what had happened in my case. To some extent I knew what went wrong, though I still did not know *why* it had happened, or had been allowed to happen. At least I had the acknowledgement of the settlement. I could sleep a little easier at night knowing that some level of justice had been served, and that my family would be provided for if I died, but I couldn't stop thinking of those other women. The thought of the document, the spreadsheet that my lawyers had been sent, which had the other women's names on it blacked out, kept flashing through my mind.

I stayed awake thinking about it. I wondered who they were and what they were doing at that very moment. How much time did they have left? I hoped they were still alive. They deserved the truth too, and so did their families. I felt a part of that dark secret. I could feel the ticking clock and the urgency for them to have the answers they deserved.

It was a whirlwind few days that followed the court case.

The story had made all the headlines. I was receiving a lot of calls and texts from journalists wanting to cover the story. I agreed to speak to the media, as much as I was able to, though I was still feeling very weak. I knew the importance of making sure the issue wasn't swept under the carpet. It was the reason I had chosen to go public. There were other women out there who had been affected the same way I had and they needed to be told.

My phone rang. I suspected it was another journalist getting in touch. It wasn't. It was the minister for health, Simon Harris. He was very apologetic and sincere. He promised me that he would do whatever he could to get to the bottom of what had happened.

The government was coming under increasing pressure to answer questions about the CervicalCheck programme. True to his word, Simon Harris announced that he would be taking immediate action. He would write to all the doctors of the women who may have been affected by the audit to make sure they had informed their patients of the result. 'It's absolutely essential that we establish that those doctors told their patients of the outcomes of those audits. We can't just presume they did, or expect or hope that they did, we have to make absolutely sure that they did, so that women can have absolute confidence in relation to that,' he said.

He also addressed me personally. 'My thoughts are with her in this most horrific and difficult time ...' he said. 'I want her to know, as Minister for Health, I don't just apologise in the role that I hold, I want to take action to make sure that we learn from it as a system.'

In the Dáil during Leaders' Questions the tánaiste Simon Coveney was also questioned on the issue. The pressure was mounting. It had hit a nerve across the country. No one could believe what had happened and how it could have been allowed to happen. The issue dominated the airwaves – politicians were being pressed for answers by journalists. They were firefighting, struggling to keep up with the revelations. I wondered if it might actually bring down the government. They needed to take action, and quickly.

Later that day, Minister Harris met with the HSE director general Tony O'Brien. They agreed that an international peer review of the CervicalCheck programme should take place 'in order to ensure ongoing confidence in the programme' as a 'matter of urgency'. This was vital. The screening programme was there for a reason, and it did save lives. It was important that women knew that they could trust it.

The HSE had released a statement around the time of the court case, saying that while the National Cervical Screening Programme is committed to providing the best possible service to women in Ireland, it is 'clearly of utmost importance to acknowledge the significant impact of this case on the client and her family'.

It said cervical screening could not prevent all cancers, and while regular screening can detect pre-cancerous changes early, '... screening tests are not diagnostic in nature and cannot always indicate the presence or absence of pre-cancerous changes ... Despite this, cervical screening represents one of the most effective ways to prevent cervical cancer.'

The statement continued: 'CervicalCheck has detected and treated over 50,000 pre-cancerous changes in women, reducing their risk of cervical cancer by more than 90%.

Figures from National Cancer Registry Ireland show that the cervical cancer rate in Ireland has reduced significantly as a direct result of the CervicalCheck programme. Despite these achievements, every diagnosis of cervical cancer is one too many and we acknowledge the impact of this disease on women and their families.'

It was all moving so fast; it was hard to keep up with what was happening. The issue seemed to be bigger than we realised. We could never have imagined though just how deep the scandal ran, and how many lives were affected. No one could ever have imagined that.

With all the uncertainty, women across the country had lost faith in the screening system. The minister took to Twitter to announce his intention to offer free repeat smear tests to anyone who wanted some reassurance:

Have heard from many women today who have had smear tests & would like a repeat test to reassure them. Am arranging for this facility to be available & the State will meet the cost of the repeat test. Arrangements on how this will operate will be outlined next week.

He also set up a national helpline for women who were worried about their smear test.

The next day, Friday – the end of a busy week – news broke that the HSE had announced that the number involved in the audit was 1,482. Therefore, the number of women affected could in fact be a great deal higher than any of us had previously thought. At this point they believed that 208 women had their smear tests audited and may have been misdiagnosed. I couldn't believe it. We always assumed it was more than a few cases, but we could never have imagined that so many women could potentially have been affected.

The issue dominated the news headlines again. Minister Harris was on *Six One News*. I turned on the TV and watched with great interest. He was talking about me.

Like the rest of the country when I heard Vicky on the steps of the courts say that she wanted to see some good come out of her horrific situation I took a number of steps ... Women who are watching this programme tonight, who have cervical cancer and are worried – 'Could I have been told earlier?' 'Was I not informed?' – they will be hearing in the early days of next week of an appointment to meet with their clinician.

I felt a chill run up my spine when he said those words. I thought of the conversation with my doctor, when I was told. I thought of all the women who would receive those calls in the next few days, who would finally know the truth. I could feel the pain they were about to feel. This was a sacred time before their lives would be changed forever.

I tried to imagine what would have come to pass if I had signed the confidentiality agreement. None of this would be happening. I felt incredibly grateful for that decision. Sometimes in life it is hard to know if you are doing the right thing. I had wondered if it was the right thing for me, for my family, to put them in the spotlight in this way, but in that moment, I knew that I had made the right decision in going public. It really mattered.

I couldn't believe how quickly things were happening. The following evening I was on *The Ray D'Arcy Show* on RTÉ television telling my story when news came through that the head of CervicalCheck, Dr Grainne Flannelly, had announced her resignation. They told me live on air. I was glad to see that things were happening as a result of my decision to go public and call for an investigation into CervicalCheck.

In Flannelly's resignation statement she said: 'I am sorry that recent events caused distress and worry to women. I have decided to step aside to allow the programme to continue its important work. I would like to take this opportunity to thank each and every one of the doctors, nurses and programme staff of CervicalCheck for their continued hard work and commitment towards delivering a first-class service for the women of Ireland.'

The HSE formally thanked Grainne Flannelly for her 'enormous dedication, contribution and expert knowledge'. They said she had helped to introduce a programme that has saved the lives of countless women in Ireland through screening and early intervention and who would otherwise have died from cervical cancer.

By the end of the weekend, the helpline had received three thousand calls.

Taoiseach Leo Varadkar spoke in the Dáil on the issue. He said he was 'full of sorrow' and 'very angry' that women were not told earlier about their smear tests being reviewed and he confirmed that an inquiry into the scandal would take place. However, he was careful to emphasise that 'cancer screening works', in order to reassure women around the country to continue to engage with the cancer screening programme.

It was Tuesday, the first of May: May Day ... Hundreds of years ago, in May, Ireland would have been alight with bonfires burning through the night to welcome in new life, a new season. As the number of women affected by the scandal was rising, I imagined the human lives being extinguished around the country by this terrible cancer, their fires going out. I could feel a burning need in me rising. We had to do something; this required urgent change. I had been invited onto *Prime Time* on RTÉ television to talk about the scandal. This was my chance.

A car arrived to collect me at my home. I felt nervous about going on the programme. At this point I wasn't used to media interviews and being in the spotlight. I sat in the back of the car and rang a friend of mine who is a lecturer in politics. We talked a little and he gave me some advice. I put down the phone and a few minutes later it rang again. It was a Dublin number. I thought it was RTÉ checking to see if I was on the way up to them.

'Hello?' I said.

'Hello,' said the voice on the other side of the phone.

It was an official from the taoiseach's office. I was taken aback; I wasn't expecting a call. He told me that the taoiseach wanted to meet with me to discuss the issue of CervicalCheck. This was the first contact I'd had with the taoiseach. The timing seemed opportune – as I was on the way to speak on *Prime Time*. I thanked him and said that in principle I would like to meet but that I had a lot of treatments coming up and would be concentrating on my health. He reiterated that the taoiseach had an open door, whenever it suited me to meet. I made a mental note. I would wait until the right moment, when I could have the most impact, and I would meet him then.

On *Prime Time* that evening I told Miriam O'Callaghan about the call. I spoke my mind on the programme. I spoke from the heart. I was frustrated. I felt the government was not doing enough to find out who was responsible for this debacle. Meanwhile, precious time was ticking by – we needed answers, and we needed them now.

On Tuesday, 8 May the government announced officially that it was establishing a scoping inquiry into the CervicalCheck screening programme. They were appointing an independent expert, Dr Gabriel Scally, to conduct the inquiry. He had a distinguished career as a senior public health doctor and advisor with the UK Department of Health. Dr Scally would report back to the minister for health by the end of the month, setting out his findings.

Simon Harris had told me about this development. We had kept in touch, and were continuing to brief one another. I felt he was on my side through it all. I trusted him, and I could see he was following through on his promises. It would later emerge that he instigated the inquiry despite the fact that his own department was against it.

He made the announcement publicly:

I gave a commitment that some good would come from this situation and today cabinet has agreed to establish a scoping inquiry into the issues which have recently come to light in relation to the CervicalCheck screening programme. We need to examine the facts and get answers quickly for Irish women, while also identifying issues that may merit a further full statutory investigation.

… I would like to acknowledge again the tireless efforts of Vicky Phelan. I have briefed her on these developments and I understand that Dr Scally has already spoken with her and will meet with her shortly.

I met with Gabriel the following day. He had called me to see if it would suit me to meet with him. He was adamant that he wanted to meet me before he started work on the inquiry, to get my sense of what needed to happen and how I felt about it. I was due at St Vincent's Hospital in Dublin for my treatment and Gabriel wanted to facilitate me. He booked a meeting room on the ward where I was having treatment and ordered teas, coffees and sandwiches. Jim had travelled up with me as this was only my second infusion of Pembro. Because I'd had such a severe reaction to the first infusion I had asked Dr Fennelly to book me in to the hospital for the night in case I had a similar reaction. Jim was going to stay at a hotel close by.

When I met with Gabriel, he said that he would do his best to get to the heart of what had happened. He explained his background and told me about a case that had just finished in Belfast which involved the deaths of five babies from hyponatraemia and in which Gabriel testified against some of the doctors he had trained with. I think he told me this story to let me know the kind of man he is, that he is principled and that he would do what he believed was right. He said that he would keep me informed at all stages of the inquiry and asked if it would be okay to call me from time to time if he had any queries.

From that day on, we kept in very close contact. I had confidence in his judgement and his resolve to get answers while at the same time trying to ensure that we still had a screening programme that worked and could be trusted.

A few days later, one of the other women affected by the scandal spoke to the media.

Suddenly, they were no longer blacked-out names on a spreadsheet – they were real people, people who now knew the truth about what had happened to them too. She spoke to Audrey Carville, the presenter of *Morning Ireland* on RTÉ Radio 1. I was standing in my kitchen, listening to the radio.

Her name was Emma Mhic Mhathúna. She was thirty-seven years old and the mother of five children. The interview brought the country to a standstill.

I learned this week that I'm dying and that the cancer is discovered in my bones and everything, so I have a test on Friday to see exactly how long I've left.

And who told you this devastating news?

My GP.

And Emma, did you think you'd be clear, did you hope you'd be clear?

I hoped I'd be clear, but I had a feeling that I was … I had a feeling I had cancer again, because I'd had it before. But I didn't think it would be terminal.

Have you told your children?

I have, yeah.

And how are they? You've a very young family.

Devastated. I'm crying thinking about it. It was the hardest thing I've ever had to do, because as a mother it's my job to protect them and to keep the bad news away from them. And we'd such a good day on the confirmation, like, my results were ready on Tuesday but I didn't want to get them because it was their confirmation. And then I had to collect them from school early and tell them that I'm dying and it's just a horrible thing to witness, to be honest, there's so much pain in the house.

Is there any treatment, anything left that you can do?

They'll know more when they get the results on Friday. But all the doctors, the gynaecologist, the oncologist, my GP ... I've such a fabulous team, I'm in good care in that sense, you know? So if there's anything available they'll find it.

And Emma, you had just found out that you had a smear test in 2013 which you thought was normal, but it wasn't, but you never knew that?

No. No. The 2013 smear said that I was healthy, when I wasn't. And because of that then I actually developed cancer. And now I'm dying. And if the smear test was right, and I was told this by my gynaecologist – who is over three hospitals, so he knows his stuff, this guy is amazing – he told me himself that if my smear test was right in 2013 I wouldn't be where I am today.

And this is what makes it so heart-breaking. I'm dying when I don't need to die. And my children are going to be without me, and I'm going to be without them. I tried to do everything right, by, you know, breastfeeding, and being a full-time mum, and sacrificing, you know, my own life for them. I didn't see it as a sacrifice and now I'm going to miss out. And I don't even know if my little baby is going to remember me.

And what just makes this whole situation so sick is that the government aren't doing anything about it. And when it first broke out I was like, 'Okay, well, the head of the HSE is surely going to do something,' and he didn't. And then

I looked to Simon Harris, I was thinking, 'Well, surely the minister for health is going to step in and do something,' that's why we give these people powers, and he didn't do anything. So then I was like, 'Surely the taoiseach is going to do something.' And he just seems to be sticking up for them. And they're all hiding there in the Dáil and they don't see what I see.

And there's women that are dead and they're not just any women, they're people's daughters and they're mammies and all the children are in so much pain. And my stance on it is I think the only person that can do something on it now is the president, and I never actually thought I'd say something like that in a country ... in 2018 ... in Ireland. Because the government need to go, they're not actually – and I'm not being insulting, it's genuine – they're not actually capable of minding us, and that is their job. To make sure that we're okay.

I'm dying and I didn't even need to die, and I'm only thirty-seven. Last night I was in bed and I was having this really bad dream. I dreamt that I was dying last night and I wasn't ready because I hadn't said goodbye to my children and in my dream I was trying to ring 999 but I couldn't pick up the phone. So in my dream I had gone in to Natasha, she sleeps across the landing, and I was trying to wake her up so that I could say goodbye to her because I hadn't said goodbye. And then I woke up and I was like, 'Thank God I haven't died yet because I want to say goodbye to them.' And this isn't fair. And no amount of money can replace this. I know which of my children like butter, and which of them need time out when they're getting tired, and all the fun stuff we do together. We have such good fun, the six of us.

And I moved all the way down here to Ballydavid because it's such a fantastic place, and all my children are boys and it's really like Enid Blyton down here; they go climbing on the rocks and they go camping in the fields and they're so safe, and they build sandcastles, and that's all being taken away from them. And yesterday I had to sit down with the teachers and I was like, 'What are we going to do?'

I was rooted to the spot. The tears were streaming down my cheeks. To hear those words coming from another woman, another mother, who was going through the same thing that I went through, broke my heart. I could feel everything that she was feeling – the worry, the pain, the anxiety. I could only hope that her prognosis would be better than mine, that she would live to see her five children grow up.

It made me angry to think that other women had to carry this needless pain. Why did they have to go through it? We should all have been spared this threat to our lives, to our families. It was all starting to feel very, very real.

It later emerged that 162 women with cervical cancer hadn't been informed about the CervicalCheck audit results. Of 209 women who could have had earlier intervention in light of false tests, eighteen had died.

I received a message from a friend of mine. She knew the husband of one of the women who had died and he had asked her if it would be okay to contact me. 'Of course,' I said.

He gave me a call. His name was Stephen Teap. His story was also heart-breaking. His wife Irene had died less than a year ago, leaving behind Stephen and their two young sons Noah and Oscar. Irene died before the truth had come out about the audit. Stephen had received the call to tell him the news that Irene was one of the eighteen women. He thanked me for all I had done. Otherwise, he said, they would never have known the truth. A note would have been made on her file, and he would never have been told.

He wanted to do something to help, he told me. Anything. He said that when the boys grew up they would learn about the scandal, and would know that their mother had been one of the women affected. 'When they ask me, "What did you do, Daddy?" he said, 'I want to be able to tell them that I did everything I could to make sure their mother's death was not in vain.'

I listened to him speaking about Irene. I could tell his heart was broken. I couldn't imagine his pain. At least I would not be the one left behind, I thought. I wasn't sure what was worse: to die, or to be left behind.

We both felt passionately that we needed to do everything we could to find the answers the women of Ireland deserved. We promised to stay in touch and to work together to see what we could do to move things forward, to change the system to make sure this could never happen again. We still had no clear explanation for why this had happened; so far, no one had taken responsibility. We were hopeful that the Scally Report would provide the answers and recommendations needed to bring about effective change.

Stephen began to tell his story to the media, to reveal what had happened to Irene and the impact it had had on his family. A few weeks later we were both invited to the Oireachtas Public Accounts Committee (PAC) by Alan Kelly, the health spokesman for the Labour Party, to speak on the issue. It would be attended by senior politicians. This was our chance to speak to the people who had the power to change things.

Stephen and I kept in touch by phone, on a daily basis. So although we had become acquainted in a short space of time, we had yet to meet in person. We arranged to meet on the train to Dublin, so that we could travel together to the Oireachtas committee hearing.

I was travelling from Limerick and Stephen was travelling from Cork. I made sure to book myself onto the train that would join the Cork to Dublin train that Stephen would be on. He had texted me the carriage number, and as I walked through the carriage, searching people's faces, I spotted him. He stood up. He had kept a seat for me.

'Stephen!' I was immediately struck by how young he was. We hugged and I sat down beside him. It was great to finally meet in person. It felt like we had known one another for a long time. We understood each other, in a way not many people could.

We talked the whole way up. It felt very natural. I hated to think of how much pain he had already experienced at such a young age. He told me about Noah and Oscar and how they were coping since their mum had passed away. He worried whether Oscar would remember his mum in years to come, he was so young. I told him all about Amelia and Darragh. I felt immediately connected to him and his family and all they had been through. I only wished I could do something to take his pain away. We both agreed that this campaign for change was what we needed. We would set our minds to working towards something positive coming out of all of this, for the sake of our children.

I wanted to make sure my daughter would be safe in the

world, to ensure that the same thing could never happen to her, or to her children, in the future. He wanted to make sure his sons lived in a world where they knew their mother had not died in vain. We needed to show our children that you could have the power to do what was right, to stand up for what you believed in, no matter how hard that would be.

We were meeting Cian, my solicitor, at Buswell's Hotel in Dublin. Across the road from Leinster House, Buswell's has been frequented by politicians for generations. We had lunch there and Stephen decided to go outside to have a cigarette to calm his nerves before we headed over to the committee meeting. He was back in less than a minute, laughing. He was just about to light his cigarette when he noticed a bunch of people racing across the road with cameras and tripods. It was the media. They had spotted Stephen and wanted a photo and an interview. This was all new for him. Cian said that he had noticed a large crowd gathering at Leinster House when he was coming in to meet us. It was all very surreal. We weren't used to photographers and media scrums. I was still surprised by it. I was just an ordinary woman. I simply told the truth and wanted others to know the truth.

A short time later we found ourselves sitting in front of a row of politicians at the Public Accounts Committee. Me, Stephen, and my solicitor Cian.

I was invited to speak first. I cleared my throat. 'If I do die, I want it not to be in vain. I want protocols to be put in place and sanctions for people who make mistakes and that the HSE is overhauled from the ground up, so that people are held accountable and that this will never happen again,' I said.

I told them my story, from the beginning, and everything that had happened over the course of the past year. 'The misdiagnosis in my case has cost me my life. I've got terminal cancer,' I said. I took a deep breath. 'I don't believe I'm going to die but I have to fight for my life every day.'

I outlined three issues that needed to be addressed: open disclosure (how could it be left up to individual doctors to decide whether or not to communicate information to their patients?), patient safety (we needed to rebuild trust in the system, to ensure this would never happen again) and responsibility of senior HSE management who approved the communication strategy regarding the audit results and whether patients were to be told about them (who was ultimately responsible for what had happened?).

'At least I'm still here to tell the tale and that's why I'm fighting with everything in my being ... I swear to God, over my dead body I'm going to keep at this. Simple as that.'

Cian O'Carroll, my solicitor, spoke of the 'coordinated, premeditated plan to deny patients the information'. 'Not in total,' he added. 'The documentation suggests that it was envisaged that some patients would be told of the audit, albeit quite late in the day.'

When Stephen spoke he emphasised the need for accountability. He couldn't understand how people in senior positions in the HSE had known about the audits and not ensured the information was communicated to the patients. Mandatory open disclosure was worthless, he said, unless sanctions were also introduced to ensure people complied with it. It didn't make sense. Patient care needed to be the backbone of the HSE. He spelled out what had happened as a result of a failed system: 'We have dead women, terminal diagnoses, death sentences.' The room was silent for a moment while everyone took in what he was saying.

He talked about his wife Irene and the life they had built together. When she became very sick her goal was to see their eldest son start school in September. She didn't make it. She died on 26 July, a few weeks before the start of the school year. She was thirty-five years of age.

Our message was clear: something had to be done.

The members of the Public Accounts Committee applauded when we had finished speaking. I could see that some had become emotional during our speeches. Fianna Fáil TD Seán Fleming, chairman of the PAC, said it was 'a deeply humbling experience' and thanked us for our 'harrowing' accounts. 'We've listened to failures of the state and state institutions and everything will be in vain if there's no fundamental changes in the future,' he said.

Meanwhile, the helpline had received 18,623 calls by then: women from all across the country worried about their smear tests and whether they too could be one of those affected.

Some days later, a text came through telling me to turn on the television, quick. I flicked on the TV and there on the news was Emma Mhic Mhathúna, the woman who had spoken out on the radio about being one of those from the audit who was misdiagnosed. I thought of the interview she had given on *Morning Ireland*, and how worried she was for her five children. The footage showed the president visiting Emma's house in Kerry. He was there to show her his support.

Tears filled my eyes as I saw the presidential car pulling up to her door and Michael D. Higgins greeting her. The country was taking this seriously, even if the health service weren't, or at least that's how it felt.

Emma Mhic Mhathúna had gone to court as well. She had settled her case against the Health Service Executive and a US laboratory for 7.5 million euro. I'll never forget the day she stood outside the courthouse, on the very spot where I had stood some months before. She was wearing a vibrant red dress chosen by her children. She said red was a symbol for standing with women. 'Whether I'm dying or not, justice is the priority here ...'

Those who had been so brutally affected by this scandal were standing strong together. The women and men of Ireland.

38

Staying Alive

'WOULD YOU NOT GIVE IT a go?' my brother said to me one afternoon as we were having a cup of tea. 'His name is Billy Watson, from Wexford. He's supposed to be very good.'

My brother was trying to convince me to go to a healer. I looked at him in disbelief. I was sceptical.

Eventually he wore me down. 'Okay,' I said. 'I'll try it.' When you're desperate, you'll try anything once.

So the following week I headed off in the car, bright and early, bound for Wexford, with Susan and Maria tagging along for reinforcement in case I needed help with anything along the way, though it may have been curiosity that was the motivating factor. We were all very curious. None of us had ever been to a healer before.

Billy was a farmer, you see. But he healed on Sundays. He learned the healing from his father, who was a seventh son, and I think his father before that.

We arrived at the farmhouse, a little place off a quiet country road. It had all the hallmarks of a working farm, with tractors and chickens in the yard. We knocked on the door. No answer. We waited a little longer and Susan knocked again. 'Hello, Billy?' she called. I started to wonder if we'd gone a little bit mad. What were we doing here, in the middle of nowhere, waiting for a healer named Billy?

A few moments later, Billy arrived, up from the field in his wellies. He welcomed us inside.

The way it works is, he heals people with the sap of the buttercup. We went in and sat down and told him about my ailments. He spoke with me for a few minutes, then went out into the garden. We watched him out the window, cutting down branches. Soon he returned. He had asked me to bring my own towels, which I now placed on the table in front of me.

Billy started a process of mashing up the sap. He put the kettle on and when it was boiled he mixed the sap with the hot water. He told me to rub the sap on the part of the body where my particular ailment was. In my case, my tumours were growing in my abdominal area. I also had a small one on my shoulder.

An hour later, we were getting back into the car. We sat in, and Susan and Maria looked at me, covered in green sap. All three of us burst out laughing. 'You never know,' I said. 'It just might do the trick.'

I visited Billy a few more times after that. I'll never know if the healing sap had any effect on me. But I won't rule anything out. I thought of my promise to Amelia and Darragh. I decided I would do anything I could to stay alive. I was willing to try anything, in addition to my medical treatment, if it helped to improve my quality of life and to allow me to live even a little bit longer.

And everyone was getting behind me. It helped a lot, to know that so many people were there with you – that nothing was too out of bounds. Friends and family were even growing the occasional cannabis plant for me in their kitchens. I used the resin to make suppositories, to give me some relief from pain. I felt like I was in an episode of *Breaking Bad*. Little did my two children know, as they were upstairs sleeping soundly in their beds, that I was downstairs turning cannabis into suppositories. It's funny the places life takes you sometimes.

The Pembro was making me stronger already. I could feel the difference in my body, but there had to be more I could do to fight this disease. I researched all the possibilities, and no matter how crazy it sounded, I was willing to try it.

And so I began my quest: visiting a bioenergy healer, going for vitamin C infusions and getting oxygen therapy – anything that might help to keep my mind and body strong. When I started visiting the bioenergy healer, Michael O'Doherty, it took a little while to get used to, but it soon became something of a lifeline for me.

The first time I went to visit him I didn't know what to expect. After we had our initial introductions, the therapy began. He stood in front of me and put his hands out, but didn't actually touch me. He explained that he was moving the energy around, drawing the negative energy out of me. Then I lay down on a bed and he did a sweep of the energy over my body. He then put on some meditative music and left the room while I lay there for half an hour.

The idea is that he works on building your positive energy. We came up with a script and I recorded myself saying it over and over again. Then he put it to music. When I got home I listened to the recording three or four times a day. It was like a mantra and I would listen to it wherever I was.

I drove to Doughmore beach in Doonbeg, my favourite place, and walked along the strand. There's a place I like to go, and sit among the rocks, and watch the waves crashing in to the shore. I sat there and recited my mantra. I closed my eyes. I could feel the cool sea breeze across my face. This was living. I couldn't imagine death. Is it the opposite of this? The mantra helped to clear the thoughts from my mind and focus on the task at hand – to stay positive and keep going.

I repeated the mantra over and over again, whenever I was in the car, or in the kitchen.

Michael has never told me he can cure cancer, or anything to that effect. I knew it wasn't about that. It's about getting your mind in the right place. Michael wouldn't accept any money from me because he said I had done so much for the women of Ireland. I persisted, but he insisted. I liked going to him. It was a bit like reiki. A kind of complementary therapy.

I trusted him. On the days I was finding things tough, his help was the support I needed to stay positive. He has worked with a lot of high-profile people. Over the months that followed there were many times I needed to maintain positive mental energy, and it helped me to stay strong during the campaign. There were numerous media interviews, television debates and newspaper articles. It could be hard to summon the energy to do it all. I found myself going back to Michael again and again.

Then I began going for vitamin C infusions at Dr Stewart's Clinic. I had researched this a lot before deciding to sign up. I found that many clinical studies have been carried out which show that it can help to improve symptoms and prolong survival in terminal cancer patients as an adjunctive part of their palliative care treatment. It can also improve energy levels and can lessen fatigue, and it has been shown to decrease pain. It was something I wanted to try. I would have to travel to Portlaoise for the infusion. When I arrived for my first appointment, the building looked like an apartment block set on top of shops and offices. I wondered if I was in the right place.

I pressed the buzzer. A voice answered. 'Yes? Who is it?'

'Vicky Phelan, here for a vitamin C infusion,' I said. I chuckled to myself. It would be a strange thing to announce if it was the wrong address.

'Come in,' said the woman on the intercom.

I went in not knowing what to expect and found myself in a room full of recliner armchairs. It reminded me of the week of my court case – all the time I had spent in the recliner. There were other people who mostly looked like cancer patients sitting in the chairs, with blankets around them to stay warm and comfortable. They were all of different ages. Some had lost their hair; others were at the start of their cancer journey.

The woman at the desk, Shannyn, checked me in and showed me to one of the chairs. The whole process would take a few hours, so it was important I made myself comfortable, propped up with cushions and blankets to stay warm. I lay back in the chair and she attached an I-V drip to my arm to allow the vitamin C to move through my body.

At the end of the session, they told me I would probably be a bit tired for a day or two, but overall, the vitamin C should give me more energy. As the days wore on, I did indeed feel more energised, and from then on I would make the journey back to Portlaoise as often as I could, to keep my vitamin C levels topped up.

The other thing I wanted to try was hyperbaric oxygen therapy.

I found a clinic in Galway, Oxygeneration, that administered it. I researched how it was supposed to work. Lots of trials had been conducted on hyperbaric oxygen's use as a cancer treatment, often with mixed or inconclusive results. In 2015, scientists in Boston made headlines with a study that concluded flooding tumours with oxygen may help some therapies work better. I decided that it was worth a try since it is used in many hospitals as an adjunct to radiotherapy to help reduce the risk of developing some of that treatment's dreaded side-effects. There is a high risk of serious complications developing after radiotherapy. In my own case, I had received the maximum dose of twenty-eight sessions of external beam radiation, as well as three doses of brachytherapy, which is internal radiotherapy. Both of these treatments make the vagina narrower, less able to stretch, and can make having sex extremely painful. If I ever wanted to try to enjoy sex again, I felt that trying out hyperbaric oxygen therapy was worth a shot.

I travelled to the clinic in Galway. When I arrived, I was shown to an oxygen chamber. It looked very futuristic. I sat in the chamber breathing in the oxygen for an hour or two. It was a strange feeling, to concentrate on breathing; we do it so often without thinking about it. It slowed everything down. It was time to sit and breathe and think.

Whenever I went for the oxygen and vitamin C infusions I tried to visualise it working against my cancer. If you read enough about cancer – and I have read a lot about cancer – there are a lot of alternative treatments available.

These kinds of therapies aren't for everyone, but for me, they acted as a complementary therapy to my medical treatment. Mentally and physically they made me feel like I had some control over things, that I could be proactive. I could get in the car and drive out to access complementary treatments that might help my chances. I was strong enough to be able to do that now. I needed to feel like I was doing all I could to keep my promise to Amelia. When you have cancer, you'll do anything you can to increase your chances of survival, and I believe it should be everyone's choice to do that if they wish. After all, it is your life, and your potential death, that is at stake.

Initially I found it difficult to visualise what my tumour looked like – to think that it is a part of my body that is trying to kill other parts of my body. My tumour is wrapped around my para-aortic lymph nodes. It nearly touches all my vital organs. It is a 10-centimetre tumour mass, if it got any bigger it would be touching off my kidneys, my heart and my liver. It stays dangerously close to all my major organs, threatening at any moment to win the battle. That was why I had come so close to dying. I never wanted that to happen again.

With help from Michael and from reading books by Joe Dispenza and other authors who believe in the power of the mind, I have come to vividly visualise my tumours. I actively visualise them disappearing, and I visualise myself as happy and healthy. My aunt Tina, who has the gift of seeing things before they happen, told me that she saw me standing on the Golden Gate Bridge in San Francisco in 2025. That is an image I like to visualise and one that I hold on to, daily.

As the months went by, I felt stronger and stronger. The Pembro seemed to be working for me. And all the alternative treatments were helping to keep me mentally strong. The life was coming back into my cheeks and I was starting to feel like myself again.

39

Letters

IT IS NOT OFTEN IN my life that dreams have come true. Mostly, life has been hard, but the day I got a call from the president of the University of Limerick, Dr Des Fitzgerald, inviting me to come and see him, I had a feeling that this might just be the makings of a lifelong dream, finally realised.

He welcomed me into his office. I pulled up a seat at his desk. He began by talking about all the work that I had done to bring the CervicalCheck issue to light, and how much it meant to the university to have me as an alumni, as a role model for the other students.

I could sense where this was going, or at least I hoped I could. If I was right, it would be one of the best things that had ever happened to me. The suspense was too much. I cut across him. 'Are you about to offer me an honorary doctorate?' I blurted out.

He laughed. 'Well, I was just about to get there ... but yes, that's exactly what I was going to do.'

'Yes!' I said. 'Yes, yes, yes!' I could not contain my excitement. Ever since I had applied for the PhD, all those years ago, before all the trauma of my illness and Amelia's accident, I had carried the weight of not having accomplished what I set out to do. Not having completed the PhD was my biggest regret in life.

An honorary doctorate would mean so much. It would be a lifelong dream fulfilled and a potential life regret wiped out at the same time. We set the date for the ceremony – 26 June. I thanked him profusely for the honour and told him how much my family and I would be looking forward to it.

Dr Fitzgerald walked me out of his office, and down the grand old staircase of what the university called the White House, as he accompanied me to the door of the building. I could see a group of people gathered at the foot of the stairs. One of them was facing the other way but looked very familiar.

'Is that Paul O'Connell, the rugby player?' I asked.

'It is,' said Dr Fitzgerald. He explained that the people who were gathered there were all part of the University Foundation. Just then, I spotted another person I recognised.

'And is that Mary Harney?' I asked, though I knew the answer.

'Yes,' he said. 'She's the chancellor of the university.'

My heart fell. I suddenly felt very torn. The chancellor would likely be presenting me with the honorary doctorate. I didn't know if I would feel comfortable accepting the doctorate from a former minister for health, who presided over the original outsourcing of smear testing in Ireland. The irony of it would be too much for me.

I had met Dr David Gibbons during one of my trips to St Vincent's Hospital for treatment. Dr Gibbons was one of the senior cytopathologists who resigned in 2008 over the government's decision to outsource smear testing. He eerily predicted that outsourcing to the United States would miss up to a thousand cases of cervical cancer over a ten-year period. I had read the coverage of the issue online. And I stood with Dr Gibbons.

I had always dreamed of having a doctorate, but I wasn't sure if this was the right way for it to happen. I decided not to voice my concerns to Dr Fitzgerald. I would go home and think it through, and get in touch with the university once I had made my decision. I imagined the photograph – me in a hat with a scroll, shaking hands with the former minister for health. Given that the reason I was receiving the doctorate was because I had been failed by the health service, it just wouldn't seem right.

I worried about what I should do, or if I was over-reacting. I talked it through with friends who worked in academia. How was I going to tell the university that I could not accept the doctorate? I was just summoning up the courage to call them when a letter arrived in the post. It was from the university. I opened it and saw the name at the bottom. I couldn't believe it. It was a handwritten letter from Mary Harney. In it she congratulated me on my work. She said she could not remember a time in the recent past when the entire population had felt more empowered by the actions and voice of one woman, whose name they did not know a few months ago. She said she knew that many felt that I had become their voice, and others felt that I enabled them to find their own voice. She said this was true of people who have issues with CervicalCheck and the health service, but that I had also instilled strength and courage in women and men who face adversity in other areas of life.

She was writing to tell me that unfortunately she would be unable to attend the conferring ceremony as she would be in

Brussels for two days at meetings at the time. She congratulated me on the award and sent every good wish for me and my family.

I breathed a sigh of relief. I could now accept the award. I would be going to the University of Limerick on 26 June to receive my doctorate after all.

On the day of the conferring I arrived at the university full of excitement. Jim was with me, as were Darragh and my parents. Amelia made the decision to be with her classmates that day; they were putting on a show as it was their last day in primary school. I totally understood; it was an important day for Amelia too. We picked her up after the ceremony and she spent the rest of the evening with us as a family.

Many other friends and family had come out to support me. It was a beautiful day. The sun was shining and I felt like the world was finally sending some good luck my way.

We gathered in the hall. I was wearing the university robes and hat. Dr Des Fitzgerald took to the podium.

Good afternoon, everybody. I'm delighted to welcome you to the University of Limerick for this most special event. I would like to extend a particularly warm welcome to Vicky Phelan, to her husband Jim, and her son Darragh. Some, like Vicky Phelan, have had a major impact on people's lives, just by the way they live their lives. I've often said it's the person who honours the degree, not the degree that honours the person. Vicky, we are delighted that you have accepted to be conferred by your alma mater at the University of Limerick. You bring great honour to this university and to our community, and for this, we honour you.

It meant a huge amount to me to be receiving the award, because researching is what I love best, and a PhD is all about celebrating the power of research.

Irene was on my mind that day. Stephen was in the audience. I caught his eye from the stage and smiled over at him. He smiled back. I knew he was thinking of Irene too and how she should be sitting beside him. I saw Darragh looking up at me from the audience. I thought of Stephen's two little boys growing up without their mother. All these thoughts were going through my mind as I sat there, waiting to receive the doctorate I had always dreamed of.

Here at the University of Limerick, we aim to instil in our students the ability to reason, to solve problems, to participate as citizens, to play their part in the social and political life of this country. The conferring of a UL honorary degree embraces these ideals. It has been awarded to just a small number of women to date, including the former president of Ireland, Mary Robinson; Adi Roche and Ali Hewson, for their contribution to volunteerism; and to Catherine Day for her leadership in the European Commission, to name a few.

Vicky Phelan has had a major impact on people's lives in this most difficult and precious time in her own. Through her courage, commitment and exceptional communication skills, she is highlighting a major issue in the Irish healthcare system. During all of this, Vicky has encouraged the women of Ireland to have faith and to continue participating in the cervical screening programme. She is an inspiration to our students, our staff and our community, she has brought great honour to the university, and for this we have awarded Vicky Phelan an Honorary Doctor of Letters.

The room erupted in applause.

It was one of the happiest moments of my life. To be back where I started out in college, all those years ago. So much had happened since. I was changed, but deep down I was still the same person I had always been, right from the beginning. I was still that little girl who ran down to the River Suir; I was the girl starting her first day in university, against all the odds; I was the girl with broken wings trying to finish my degree, despite the trauma of the car accident; I was the woman who eloped to get married in St Lucia; I was the mother of a child with a serious medical condition; I was the woman who stood on the steps of the courthouse and asked for change. I was all of these things, all at once. To me the degree symbolised every part of my life, all of the love and pain along the way. That was the research of my life.

It reminded me of a song that Amelia and I sing together: 'This is Me' from the musical *The Greatest Showman*. The song is about standing up to say, 'This is me, scars and all, and I'm proud of who I am.' We both have scars to remind us of the pain we've suffered, but despite it all, or maybe because of it all, we know who we truly are. When Amelia and I are in the car alone, we turn the volume up high and sing the song at the top of our voices. When I stood up to accept the doctorate, scarred and bruised, I took a breath and smiled. This is me.

40

The Man From Cashel

I WAS STARTING TO LOOK forward to the sound of the postman – the creak of the letterbox opening and closing and the soft thud of letters landing on the mat.

One morning I woke to that familiar sound. I was feeling very tired, though I was sleeping a little better. A local Limerick company had sent me a recliner bed when they heard me speaking on the radio, which was helping me to sleep more comfortably. The excitement of seeing what had arrived in the post gave me a good reason to get up. I got dressed and headed downstairs.

The light was streaming through the house, and there on the mat was a pile of letters. I picked them up and went to the kitchen to open them over a cup of tea. Each of the envelopes was addressed in different handwriting, handwriting I didn't recognise. All except one, addressed in a way that had become very familiar to me. On it was the moniker of the hospital and the officious lettering in small black type. These were the kinds of letters that came for Mrs Victoria Phelan. They were never good news.

I put the hospital letter down on the counter, made a cup of tea, and settled myself before I opened it. It was from the consultant's secretary. It was a reminder that I was to come to the hospital for an appointment the following week to have a CT scan. This would be my first scan since I had started the Pembro infusions. My oncologist had explained that I would have a scan after every three to four infusions to allow him to see whether or not the drug was having an effect on my tumours.

I began to experience the familiar anxiety of waiting for a scan. I could feel that the drug was working. My abdomen had shrunk significantly. I was no longer wearing maternity clothes. I had more energy and was starting to feel more like myself. But with cancer, it was always so hard to know. I needed the certainty of knowing for sure that it was working, that I was really getting better. Also, if we knew that it worked, it would help us to make the argument to allow the drug to be more widely available for other women with cervical cancer. All I could do was wait.

I took a deep breath and began opening the other letters.
One was addressed:
'Vicky Phelan,
Limerick'
That was all. Somehow it had reached me.

I tore it open. It was a handwritten letter from a woman, thanking me. She said because she had heard my story, she had gone for a smear test. They had found pre-cancerous cells, and had been able to treat it quickly. I loved hearing good news. One by one I opened the envelopes. Each had a card or a handwritten letter enclosed, thanking me for what I had done, or wishing me luck and sending me thoughts and prayers.

I placed the cards along the windowsill and looked at them, trying to take it all in: the kindness of all these strangers who had taken time to write, to let me know they were on my side.

I had been getting cards and letters from people all over the country. Some were handwritten letters thanking me for what I was doing. Others were envelopes with medals enclosed, or messages saying God was the only way to cure my cancer. All kinds of people, all kinds of thoughts and prayers coming through my door. It helped me to cope. I placed the medals in a drawer with all the other things people had sent me: a pair of socks a woman had knitted for me, by hand; a set of angel wings another woman had made with my name on one side and Amelia's name on the other. I looked at the careful stitching of our names. I thought of all the time that had gone into making it. It was keeping me going. I felt like people were rooting for me, that they were behind me.

That night I went for a walk to pick up a few things from the shops. I was deep in thought, when suddenly I noticed two bright lights coming my way. The car pulled in and came to a stop beside me. It was dark out. I squinted to try and make out who was in the car, to see if it was someone I knew.

The window rolled down. I quickened my pace. 'Excuse me,' came a voice from inside the car, calling after me. 'Are you Vicky Phelan?'

I stopped. I turned and looked in the window. Inside the car were two men. The driver looked to be in his seventies, and the man in the passenger seat in his eighties.

'I am,' I said, taken aback.

They both smiled.

'Oh, thanks be to God,' said the man at the wheel. 'I've been looking for you for hours.'

'I'm Gerry,' he said, 'and this is Joe.' Joe nodded to confirm the story, looking delighted to have found me.

'Okay,' I said, curiously. 'Can I help you?'

'We were going to search all of Limerick if needs be, to try and find you,' said Gerry. 'I have something for you.'

He leaned over and carefully took something out of the glove box. It was a package, wrapped in brown paper. He held it carefully in both hands. He placed it delicately into the outstretched hands of the man in the passenger seat, who presented it to me out the window.

'There's a woman in Cashel with a relic, you see, and she wants you to have it.' He explained that the relic is usually booked out for weeks at a time and even though someone else was supposed to have it that week, the woman had wanted me to have it. And on her instruction, he had driven all the way from Cashel to deliver it safely to me.

I didn't have the heart to tell him, after him coming all this way to find me, that I wasn't really religious. I wondered what sort of relic it might be.

'Everything is explained in the piece of paper,' he said, pointing to the package. 'My number is in there too. Give me a call in a week.'

I carefully placed it inside my bag. I looked up to say thank you. He gave me a wave.

'Good luck,' he said, and drove away into the night.

There I was, on my own again, standing on the side of the road, now in possession of a relic, trying to work out what had just happened. When I got home, I went upstairs to the bedroom. I took the package out of my bag and laid it out on the bed.

There were layers and layers of wrapping. I peeled them off one by one. Then I saw it: the relic. It was a delicate frame, with a piece of cloth inside it. It looked very precious, like something that was very well loved and looked after. The small plaque on the frame explained that the cloth was from Saint Padre Pio.

I didn't feel connected to religion anymore, but at the same time, there was something about saints I could relate to. They seem more like characters and people. Padre Pio is a saint of hope and healing. He knew pain and he carried his wounds with him. The stigmata were imprinted on his body.

There was a piece of paper inside with instructions which told me to sleep with the relic close to my body for a week.

I was sceptical. It all seemed a bit bizarre. I had a week to go until my scan. I looked at the relic for a moment. It's worth a try, I said to myself. I placed it carefully under my pillow.

At the end of the week I called Gerry to give it back to him, as I was sure there must be a queue of people waiting for it, each with their own reason, their own ailment perhaps, in need of hope and healing. He collected it the following day.

I went to Dublin to have my scan. Dr Fennelly said that he would call me in a day or two with the results. But I felt distracted that day. I had other things on my mind. I was looking forward to getting back home. Something very exciting was to take place that weekend. I hadn't been this excited for as long as I could remember.

My favourite band, The Stunning, whose music I had been listening to since I was a teenager, were coming to Kilkenny to play a gig just for me. This private gig all came about when my friends and neighbours were organising a fundraising table quiz for me back in February when I was desperately trying to get onto the clinical trial in America. My friend Anita, who was organising the quiz, had contacted The Stunning through their website. She told them everything I had been through, and all about the trial. She explained what a big fan of their music I was, and how it would mean the world to me to see them, if there was any way they would be able to play for the fundraiser.

Their manager, Sasha, replied to Anita to say that the band were, unfortunately, gigging in the UK on the date of the table quiz, but that they wished me well with my fundraising efforts and with getting onto the clinical trial. Fast forward a couple of months and the band were watching the news one day, hearing about this woman called Vicky Phelan. The name sounded familiar, so they checked back over their emails, and sure enough – I was the same Vicky Phelan they had been told about.

The band's manager contacted Anita again and asked if I would get in touch with her. When I called Sasha she told me that the band were very taken with my story and were inspired by the fight that I was putting up to our government and that they wanted to play a private gig for me and my friends. Well, you could have knocked me with a feather. I was absolutely blown away. And so, the preparations began in earnest for the gig of a lifetime. The date was set for 13 June and I had invited all of my friends – my best friends, college friends, school friends, neighbours and family, all the people who had been with me every step of the way – to a top-secret night with The Stunning playing just for us.

Maria, Susan and I went into my sister Lyndsey's hair and makeup salon, to get ourselves beautified for the night. I had just had my makeup done and Lyndsey was starting on my hair. The music was booming in the background and the excitement was building. Lyndsey had just opened a bottle of bubbly to get ourselves going for later that evening, when I saw Dr Fennelly's number flashing on my mobile. I froze. Lyndsey saw the look on my face. I thought about letting it go to voicemail; I really didn't want to ruin my night if the news was bad. But then logic took over and I thought to myself that the news had to be good because I was feeling so well. So I answered the call. I stepped outside of the salon with rollers in my hair.

'Hi, Dr Fennelly,' I said.

He told me he had good news. The scan showed that there was significant shrinkage in my tumours. I asked him how significant. He told me that they had reduced by fifty per cent. I burst into tears. I couldn't believe it. 'Thank you so much for the call,' I said. 'Thank you so much, for everything! I think there is some celebrating to do tonight.'

As I walked back into the salon with tears streaming down my face, all eyes were on me. Lyndsey turned off the music. Everyone thought that the news was bad. They gathered around me. 'What did he say?' Lyndsey asked.

I could barely get the words out, I was crying so much. I burst out with a smile and said, 'It's good news, it's good news! The tumours have shrunk.'

The four of us hugged each other. They too were crying, tears of happiness. All the pent-up emotions that we were all trying to hold in for so long came pouring out. And then Colette, the makeup artist, yelled over, jokingly, that we were ruining her good work. And sure enough when we looked at each other, all we could do was laugh. There was mascara running down our faces.

I got back into the car to drive back to my parents' house to get ready for the night ahead. I sighed with relief, looked at the sky and said a little thank you to Padre Pio. Because, you never know, maybe the man from Cashel really did have something to do with it.

People are good. They are what gets you through.

The gig was in Jim's parents' pub. I walked in to see familiar faces all around me. The atmosphere was electric. Everyone was catching up, the pints were flowing and we were all just happy to be there.

The band started up and the crowd went wild. I couldn't believe this was actually happening. Since I was a teenager I had idolised The Stunning. Their music had seen me through. Their songs were like an anthem to my life.

Steve Wall, the band's lead singer, called me up to the stage. 'We believe Vicky has an announcement she would like to make ...'

I stepped onto the stage and took the microphone. There were yelps and cheers from everyone in the crowd. I thanked the band for their incredible generosity in coming to play for us in this way. I told them how much it meant to me. I also thanked everyone in the room for all the ways they had been there for me and my family.

'I also have another bit of news I'd like to share with you tonight ... I received a phone call earlier today from my oncologist. He gave me the results of my latest scan, and it is the best news I could ever have hoped to receive – my tumours have shrunk by fifty per cent!'

The crowd erupted with whoops of joy and applause. My family rushed over to hug me. I was crying again, with happiness. The band began to play in celebration. The drum symbols were crashing and the bass was strong. They played 'This Happy Girl'.

We all sang along. I closed my eyes and sang the lyrics as loudly as I could. They had new meaning to me all of a sudden.

> ... *As candles burn*
> *As voices hum*
> *As guilt from passion spills*
> *And the saints look on*
> *I cannot hide*
> *I cannot hide*
> *This happy girl*
> *This happy girl.*

It was one of the happiest moments of my life, and a memory I will treasure for the rest of my days.

41

The Other Women

I T WAS AROUND THIS TIME that the seeds for the 221+ group were planted.

It was Stephen's idea. He said that the day he was told that his wife Irene was one of the eighteen women affected by CervicalCheck, who had died. He was brought in to meet with Irene's consultant to find out more. He had been given an evening appointment, 7 p.m. There was no consideration given to the fact that Stephen was now a single parent and that he would have to get a babysitter. It was an awful meeting. There were clearly other women who had been told to come in at the same time. Everyone was distressed.

Stephen did not get home until after eleven o'clock that night. The babysitter went home and he sat there alone in his sitting room with the weight of what he had just been told. He had been sent home with no support and very few answers to his questions. He thought of all the other families who were receiving the news in a similar way and how utterly alone and bereft they must be feeling. And it was then that the idea of a support group for the women and families affected by the CervicalCheck scandal came to him.

The patient support group would represent the victims of the scandal. By now, the number of women believed to have been affected was 221, but we kept the plus after the number as we didn't know if this would increase. The audit that CervicalCheck had started was stopped in the wake of my case so we knew that there would potentially be a significant number of additional members who would join our support group once the audit was up and running again. We were still waiting for this audit to report back.

The government decided to have an independent body, the Royal College of Obstetricians and Gynaecologists (RCOG), review the remaining cases of women who had been diagnosed with cervical cancer, who had not been audited by CervicalCheck. Meanwhile, we continued to engage with Dr Gabriel Scally on any questions he had as he conducted his report. It was near completion, he told us. We waited anxiously to hear what his findings would be.

Stephen and a woman named Lorraine Walsh, who had also been affected by the CervicalCheck scandal, were nominated by Gabriel and appointed by health minister Simon Harris to a steering committee as patient representatives. The committee was tasked with providing oversight and assurance on the implementation of key decisions taken by government in relation to CervicalCheck. They were there to make sure that decisions were actioned effectively.

In order to explain what they had gone through, Stephen and Lorraine put together a piece called 'Imagine' which they read to the members of the committee.

'Imagine going home this evening and your children not being there. Imagine deleting them from your life – the moment you found out that you were going to have a baby, the moment they were born, their first cry, their first steps, their first words, the first time they said Mama or Dad. Imagine not tucking them into bed at night and reading them their favourite bedtime story.'

Lorraine continued: 'Imagine seven surgeries to try and preserve fertility and allow us to have the children we so desperately longed for, followed by failed IVF because the surgery depleted my ovarian reserve due to compromised blood supply ... Imagine over five years of our lives being consumed with pain, surgery, heartache, tears and disappointments. I don't need to imagine this; this is my life.'

Lorraine and her partner had desperately wanted a child. Lorraine was diagnosed with cancer in 2012 after a smear test. However, her smear test the previous year had come back clear. 'Had it been read properly the year before, I would have been able to have a baby,' she said. She would have avoided the surgery that made it impossible for her to have children.

On the other hand, Stephen had two children, but had lost his wife. His two boys had lost their mother. 'Imagine,' he said, 'during the night your child being sick and crying for the tender touch of his mother, trying to comfort him in his sickness while consoling him that she can't be there to hold him.' This was Stephen's reality at home. But the hardest part of all was to imagine 'that it all could have been avoided if someone had done their job properly'.

'I am blessed with a wonderful partner that Stephen longs to have back in his life,' said Lorraine, 'and Stephen is blessed with two beautiful boys that I so desperately wanted.'

'The day that Irene died or the day I found out that she could have lived, I don't know which is worse,' Stephen once said. This was something he would have to live with for the rest of his life, something we were all living with – the 'what if'.

Lorraine, Stephen and I could relate to one another, though we all had a very different experience. We were all going through pain, the deepest kind of pain, the pain of love and loss, and we all knew it could have been avoided. That was the crux of it all. That was the cross we had to bear. Us, and 218 other women and their families, across the country.

Ruth Morrissey was one of these women. She had contacted me shortly after my court case. We discovered that we lived less than a mile from one another. We soon became close friends, regularly meeting for coffee.

She and her husband Paul filed her case in the High Court, with Cian O'Carroll also acting as her solicitor. She was now terminally ill and going through treatment. It made me angry to think that another woman would have to go through what I went through – having to endure an adversarial court case, being forced to sit and give evidence, at such a difficult time in her life. The government had promised that no other woman would have to go through this. And yet here was Ruth, preparing for the same kind of battle I had faced.

I decided now was the time to use the trump card I had been so carefully holding onto – the open invitation from the taoiseach to meet. I rang the number that I had received the call from on the way to my *Prime Time* interview; I got through to the taoiseach's private secretary. I would be in Dublin the following Wednesday for treatment, I told him, and if the taoiseach was available to meet, I would like to take him up on his invitation. The main topic I wished to discuss was women from the CervicalCheck scandal being dragged through the courts.

The meeting was arranged and the following week, I made my way to Leinster House. I was greeted at the door and brought through to the taoiseach's private office. He invited me to sit down. We had a coffee and talked for fifteen to twenty minutes. Then three of his advisors arrived and that's when the serious questioning began.

I had written out a list of questions I wanted answered. I had done all my research, thoroughly – I wanted to make sure I got the most out of this meeting. We discussed several issues, including the Patient Safety Bill, but the thing I really wanted clarity on was the government's commitment to the 221 women directly affected by this scandal that they would have an alternative to the courts in their quest for answers following the wrongs that had been done to them. After a lengthy discussion, I left with what I felt was a strong assurance from the taoiseach.

I had told him what a harrowing place the courtroom was for women like me who were going through treatment for a terminal illness. He assured me that the state would try to settle all further cases being taken by women and their families affected by the scandal, through mediation. And if mediation didn't work, 'an alternative dispute resolution mechanism' would be created. Something had to be done so that women like Ruth did not have to go through this anymore. I was hopeful that they would find another mechanism for Ruth's case to be settled. It remained to be seen whether any of these promises would come to pass.

*

In a way the campaign was keeping me going – it kept me focused on something positive and meaningful. But I also wanted to make sure that I wasn't spending too much time away from my children. I wanted to put them first. It was getting difficult to juggle it all at times, between the Pembro treatments in Dublin, the alternative treatments I would travel to around the country, meetings of the steering committee for the 221+ support group, and all the media interviews – there were a lot of them these days – and public engagements.

I was being invited to give talks at different events around the country. I was honoured to be asked and I liked to do them, if I could. I felt it was a good way to keep the issue alive and to create awareness about cervical cancer. If even one young woman had a smear test because she heard me speak, and it helped her to avoid this awful illness, then it would be worthwhile.

It brought me to places I had been before – including my old school, to give a talk on the power of education. As I looked out at the students gathered in the hall I thought back to the day when I had convinced Mr Dineen to let me start school early. School had been the launch pad for everything that came afterwards. It also brought me to places I never imagined I would go – I was invited to the British ambassador's residence for the visit of Prince Harry and Meghan Markle. When I introduced myself to the new royal bride, she said she knew who I was and had been following my story. I was astounded. She told me to keep up the good work. The highlight of the evening for me, however, was meeting Mary Robinson, who told me that she admired my resolve. I told Mary that I was just a stubborn bitch. It was out of my mouth before I remembered who I was speaking to. We both burst out laughing. She said that I reminded her of her younger self, but that she preferred the term 'sophisticated bad girl'.

Often when I travelled, people recognised me. I still hadn't got used to this. In the streets they would approach me to shake my hand or thank me for what I had done for the women of Ireland. It was humbling. They would also tell me their stories – often they had experienced cancer themselves, or someone they loved had. It seemed to affect nearly every family in Ireland. I loved that people were talking about it, though. It made it less lonely, for everyone. Cancer can be hard. And it happens behind closed doors. Often it is only those closest to it that truly understand it.

I decided it was a good time to get away for a special trip with the children. I was feeling a little better, and wanted to make memories with my children and go on the holiday of a lifetime. I knew they'd love it. We sat Amelia and Darragh down in the sitting room.

'We have a surprise for you.'

'What is it?' Darragh cried out.

'Well … your dad and I … are going to take you on a special holiday to Florida! We'll even get to go to Universal Studios and go on all the rides.'

They both erupted in yelps of joy. Darragh was jumping up and down on the couch. We laughed. I took a mental photograph of that moment, wanting to store it in my memory bank. I loved seeing them happy.

I had a check-up and received the go-ahead from my oncologist. My treatment was going well, so they felt it would be safe for me to go. We managed to organise a special pass so that I could avoid the long queues. I wouldn't have been able for them.

Universal Studios was a magical place, full of colour, a dream come true for the children.

'Come see this, Mam!' they'd yell, pointing at another ride or another fairy tale character.

They convinced me and Jim to join them on some of the faster rides. In the Wizarding World of Harry Potter, we climbed aboard a ride called The Forbidden Journey. All of a sudden, we were whooshed into the air. We all let out a scream. We were getting higher and higher, until we found ourselves soaring above the grounds of Hogwarts Castle with Harry and Hermione and Ron. I felt like I was flying. I had my wings again. We were free as birds. 'Wahoooo!' yelled Amelia. We laughed and held on tight to one another's hands. Just for a moment, we were able to forget about cancer. We were just a family again.

I will treasure that moment for the rest of my life and I hope that in years to come the children will look back on those photos and remember the magic of the happy times.

42

Nuns Don't Get Cervical Cancer

A LL TOO SOON, I WAS brought back to reality. I was at home in bed. The alarm on my phone was loud and insistent. I was drifting in and out of a deep sleep. I reached over to turn it off and saw a number flashing across the screen. It was a phone call. It looked like one of the radio station numbers. It stopped ringing. Bleary-eyed, I looked at the phone – seven voicemails and ten text messages. The phone rang again. I answered.

'Hello?'

'Hi, Vicky.'

'Stephen?'

'Sorry, Vicky, you sound like you were asleep.'

'What is it? What's happened, Stephen?'

'Well, there's an article in *The Irish Times* this morning on the Scally Report.'

'How do you mean?' As we hadn't received the findings yet, I wondered how it could be out in the open for others to see.

'It's been leaked, Vicky.'

'You're fucking kidding me.'

'I wish I was!'

I was feeling nauseous. I sat up on the side of the bed. I couldn't believe it. The report we had fought for had been released without us, the victims, having read it. Stephen and I spoke for a good half an hour to strategise. He said he'd make a few enquiries and come back to me.

The phone rang again. This time it was a researcher from a radio programme to see if I would come on the show to give a reaction to the report. I explained that I hadn't seen it, that I was just waking up and I would call back once I had read through it and had time to examine its findings. It wasn't meant to go public for another few days, I explained. How could I give a reaction to something I hadn't read?

I put down the phone. I could see the stream of messages and voicemails coming in from journalists across the country, each looking for a reaction to something I hadn't seen. I got out of bed. I was feeling exhausted. The phone rang again. I picked it up. Another journalist. I explained the situation again. He sounded surprised to hear that I hadn't read it.

Who had leaked the report, I wondered. How had the Department of Health allowed this to happen? I went to the bathroom and splashed some water on my face. I wiped the sleep from my eyes and tried to prepare myself for a very different kind of day.

I had planned to sleep in, for the first time in a long time, in order to have enough energy to spend time with the children. I had been feeling ill again. I was very tired these days. Instead

I had woken up to a whitewash. The phone was ringing again.

I made myself a strong coffee and sat down at the kitchen table. I took out my laptop and googled 'Scally Report'. There it was, the *Irish Times* report. The top line read: 'A commission of investigation into the CervicalCheck controversy, as promised by the Government, is not needed, according to the Scally Report, to be published this week.' I pounded my fist on the table. After everything we'd been through, this is how we were finding out. I was livid.

Stephen called again. They had formulated a plan. Gabriel would travel to Limerick shortly by train, as would Stephen and Lorraine. We would meet in a local hotel and Gabriel would brief us on the report's findings.

I could tell they were trying to accommodate me, with everyone travelling to Limerick for the briefing. They didn't want me to have to travel to Dublin unnecessarily. My muscles were aching and I had a constant underlying feeling of nausea.

That afternoon we gathered at the hotel meeting room. Gabriel carefully took out the 200-page report and placed it on the table in front of us. This was it, what we had been waiting for: an independent inquiry into the cervical scandal. I searched his eyes for clues as to its contents. The newspaper report implied that Gabriel did not think a further investigation was justified. I hoped he was on our side with this. An investigation *was* required, and we were the proof: a woman without a child, a man without a wife, and me, soon to lose my life.

I tried to imagine the damage that it would do to everything we'd fought for if the report deemed the scandal to be less critical, or played it down in some way.

We opened it. It began:

Dear Minister

This major crisis emerged into the public domain because of a failed attempt to disclose the results of a retrospective audit to a large group of women who had, unfortunately, developed cervical cancer. In particular, it emerged because of the extraordinary determination of Vicky Phelan not to be silenced. But there are many indications that this was a system that was doomed to fail at some point. Screening services are sometimes finely balanced in terms of benefit and harm and can act as an early warning sign of wider systemic problems.

We moved through the sections, one by one, with Dr Scally reading aloud and guiding us along.

The current policy and practice in relation to open disclosure is deeply contradictory and unsatisfactory. In essence, there is no compelling requirement on clinicians to disclose. It is left up to their personal and professional judgement. I know, very well, from very many of the women themselves and the families, that the issue of non-disclosure is felt very intensely. They have expressed very clearly their anger at not being told at the time when the information from the audit became available, and they are equally as angry about how they were eventually told. In my view, the manner in which they were eventually told of their situation in many cases varied from unsatisfactory and inappropriate, to damaging, hurtful and offensive.

What I was really struck by, as we thumbed through the report, was the number of personal stories included, from people Dr Scally had spoken to: women who were still alive, and the families of those who had died – husbands, daughters and sons who had lost a woman they loved. We were all silent, trying to take everything in. It was very emotional hearing of all the ways people were hurting across the country, because of what had happened.

Dr Scally recommended that members of the medical profession needed to sit down and hear from the women who were impacted by the scandal – they needed to hear these stories.

He referred to one incident outlined in the report that 'verged on misogyny': the experience of family members of one deceased woman who said the consultant in their disclosure meetings spoke 'several times about the late woman's smoking habit and also told them that nuns don't get cervical cancer'.

I felt my temperature rise. In a country where young women have been sent to camps like the Magdalene laundries, shamed and discarded, where they have been repeatedly denied their rights, it seemed as though nothing had changed. A woman was now being blamed for getting cancer. Why? For having sex – the same way any man has sex. I felt ashamed to be Irish. It seemed like women in this country had always been something to be used and shamed. We were subhuman. The system failed us time and time again, and here we were again, in 2018, and still nothing had changed.

Five hours went by as we pored over the pages, hardly stopping for a moment, until it was dark outside. Stephen looked at his watch. He needed to catch the train, to get home to his boys, but we were still not finished reading the report. We asked Gabriel if we could take it home with us, to finish reading it overnight, so that we could fully respond the next day.

'I can't give it to you,' he said. 'I would really like to be able to, but I can't.' He explained that it was a legal document that needed to be sent to the attorney general and the Department of Health before leaving his possession.

'Who makes that ultimate decision?' I asked.

'Well, I suppose the minister does,' he said.

I took out my phone and called Simon Harris's number.

He answered quickly. 'Vicky ...'

He apologised for the leak. He sounded really genuine. I could tell he was sorry it had happened. I emphasised the irony of an investigation into poor communication with patients being leaked to the public, without being communicated with those same patients. I told him it seemed like the utmost disrespect to the women and their families. He agreed it was not a good scenario and the last thing he wanted to happen, he assured me. They were working hard to get to the bottom of how it had been leaked to the media.

I told him we needed to take the report home, because after five hours, we were still not finished. He explained that it wasn't possible. It was a legal document and it couldn't leave until it had been read by the department.

I told him it was not our fault that things had happened this way. We had to be allowed to read the report that was about us, about our lives. After all, we weren't the ones who would leak anything. Of anyone, we were the ones who could be trusted the most. This was too important to us. We needed to be able to read the report.

He was silent for a moment and then said he would call back in a few minutes. He did so, and said he'd spoken with the attorney general and that we could take the report home, but on the condition that it was not shown to anyone else.

I thanked him and put down the phone.

'There we go!' I said. 'We can take it home now.' The others looked at me in disbelief.

That night as I lay in bed, I continued reading the report. It made fifty recommendations to the government. But would any of them come to pass?

We all still needed answers and a reassurance that changes had been made. Or else we would die, one by one, without those answers or hope for the future.

43

The Toll

FOR SOME, IT WAS ALREADY too late.

I had just heard from Tony O'Reilly, the husband of one of the 221 women, that his wife Julie had died. Julie O'Reilly passed away peacefully surrounded by her family on Saturday, 6 October at St Vincent's University Hospital. She was sixty-one. I had visited Julie the previous Wednesday, when I was in Dublin for treatment. As I left the hospital that day after saying my goodbyes to Julie and to Tony, I struggled to hold it together. I was trying to remember Julie full of life and smiling, like I had known her when we met on St Anne's, the day ward where I go for treatment. I got into my car to drive home, and for a few minutes I just sat there and stared out the window. I was now acutely aware of what the inside of the End of Life suite looked like in St Vincent's. That is actually what they call it, the End of Life suite. All I knew was that I did not want to end up there. Not yet.

And now, news was breaking that Emma Mhic Mhathúna

had passed away, the day after Julie, on 7 October 2018, in Kerry University Hospital. She was only thirty-seven and left behind five young children. How quickly she went, in the end. I remembered her just a few weeks ago, standing on a platform, megaphone in hand, with her two young sons by her side, calling on the government to act.

She was a powerhouse. She was determined. And then suddenly, she was gone.

Her wish was to be brought back to her favourite place, her home in Ballydavid. There was a mass held in her local church in Séipéal na Carraige in the west Kerry Gaeltacht region where Emma had lived with her children. The church was packed to capacity. Her youngest son sat on top of his mother's coffin.

Another mass was to be held in Dublin at St Mary's Pro Cathedral. When she was a little girl, Emma and her mother would attend mass at the Pro Cathedral, which is opposite the Department of Education buildings where Emma's mother worked, and they would go to light a candle together.

I went to the mass in Dublin. I left the house that morning, and braced myself for the day ahead. Cian had agreed to accompany me. He understood how difficult this day would be. It was one of the saddest days I had ever experienced – to know that Emma's life had been taken in such a way and to see her five children left without a mother, grieving at such a young age.

That afternoon, as was her dying wish, a hearse carrying her coffin ceremoniously passed by Leinster House, the seat of the government. It came to a stop outside the wrought-iron gates and paused for a few minutes. It then passed by Government Buildings, stopping again outside the Department of Health. Then the funeral cortege made its way through the city and into the Phoenix Park, where it stopped outside Áras an Uachtaráin, the president's residence, as a mark of gratitude to President Michael D. Higgins who had visited Emma at her home in Kerry.

Her family released a statement about the funeral cortege:

The purpose of this route is not to protest ... It is a final and departing effort to encourage those within to hold a mirror up to the organisations and agencies that they preside over. Moreover, it is a request to those organisations and agencies to commit to ensure that Emma's tragic situation will never happen to another Irish mother or woman again.

Hundreds attended the funeral mass. And many more people stood solemnly along the roadside as the coffin slowly passed, giving respect to Emma and all she stood for.

That night I lay in bed, in the quiet of the night with only my thoughts for company. The images of the past few days were running through my mind. With my husband and two children tucked up in bed, I felt so very grateful to be alive and well. Yet my heart was breaking for Julie's family and for Emma's family, and all the other families affected by this cancer. This brought the death toll in the CervicalCheck scandal to twenty. I couldn't help but wonder how long it would be before it would be my own funeral, my own coffin, my own children grieving the loss of their mother. It was all so very close to home. Too close.

44

Education

THERE ARE TIMES IN LIFE when you are given the opportunity to take stock and reflect on what matters, on what has really made the difference in your life.

When I heard I was being awarded an honorary fellowship by Waterford Institute of Technology, and that they would like me to give a speech, I thought long and hard about what I might say. What had really made the difference in my life? When I thought about it, it was simple. It all came down to education. That's what mattered most.

When I took the stand to accept the award, proudly wearing the WIT robes, I decided this would be a chance to say it all – to thank the people I needed to thank for bringing me on this journey. I tended not to say things, to leave them to be said some other time, but more and more I was realising that it's important to tell people how you feel, while you have the chance to do it.

I thanked WIT for awarding me an honorary fellowship –

the highest honour they could bestow upon me. I really was honoured, especially since I had been working at WIT for the past eleven years and saw in the Literacy Development Centre the difference it was making to people's lives.

'I am a true lifelong learner,' I said. '… I pursued a career working in education because of my love of learning and my passionate belief in the power of education to change lives. It was Nelson Mandela who said education is the most powerful weapon which you can use to change the world.'

It was education that finally set me free – that gave me wings to be anything I wanted to be in the world. It was education that made it possible for me to stand up for what I believed in, to take on the authorities when everything was stacked against me. I thanked Miss Keyes, my secondary school teacher, for always believing in me. She had sent me a note when she heard I was getting the award. 'I always knew you would do something great,' she'd said. 'But I always wished that your something great would have manifested itself publicly without the pain.'

I continued with my speech: 'A debacle is an event that is a complete failure. Following the presentation of the Scally Report we now know that the CervicalCheck screening programme was doomed to fail. It failed me, it failed women and families who lost their wives, mothers, daughters, friends. It failed … [over 200] other women, who like me, were misdiagnosed, or who are now fighting to stay alive or are battling side-effects that they would not be having had their cancer been detected earlier.'

I spoke about the importance of a student going on to third-level education and how, without the training I received at third level, I would have found it difficult to do the research to make the tough decisions I had to make along the way.

I told the congregation that as I stood before them, in the

chapel in WIT, my tumours had shrunk by fifty per cent and that I had a quality of life I believed I would not have had on palliative chemotherapy.

I spoke of my wish to create an advisory role, to employ someone to be available to give advice to cancer patients and their families about the most recent research in cancer medicine and the trials available. I had seen first-hand how many people around the country desperately needed this service.

I had never known what I wanted to do 'when I grew up', I told them. 'I believe that what happened to me happened to me for a reason ... This is what I was here for. That is, to improve the lives of women, in order to eradicate this awful disease for my daughter and my daughter's generation.'

I looked at Amelia, sitting in the audience.

'The pending implementation of the fifty recommendations of the Scally Report will undoubtedly save many lives. I truly believe it.'

I ended by thanking my parents, John and Gaby, who always believed in me. I looked at them, sitting in the audience beside Amelia. I thought of all the ways they had stood by my side, like my mother teaching me how to read from a very early age. All the ways they guided me through my childhood and helped me to believe in myself. I thought of my father sitting by my side in France as I lay in my hospital bed after the car accident. I thought of all the days they helped me through my cancer, and helped me with the children. I owed everything to them. I hoped I could do them proud before I died – then my life would have been worthwhile.

I needed to see the changes in the health system, to know that my fight had been effective, so that I would die knowing that Amelia would be safe, that her generation would never have to go through anything like this again. She had been through enough in her lifetime already. If I could do one thing, I wanted to do this.

A few weeks later, I was taken by complete surprise when the BBC named me as one the world's 100 most inspiring women, in recognition of my outstanding contribution to society. It was a great honour to be named in that list of incredible women from all around the world who they described as 'leaders, trailblazers and everyday heroes'. All of the nominated women were fighting for some kind of change, to try and make some small difference in the world. I read their stories – the adversity they faced, be it in India, or Africa, or parts of Europe or America. I was in awe of these women and what they were doing. I felt very proud to be a woman and to stand alongside them.

Soon afterwards, I received a Special Recognition Award from *Irish Tatler* at their Woman of the Year Awards and was named Kilkenny Person of the Year. Both meant a great deal to me. So much had happened, in such a short space of time.

My birthday was coming up. I would be forty-four. It was hard to believe it had been a year since Eilish and I had cycled the greenway. I had lived another year. A reason to celebrate.

After our cycle, Eilish and I had made a pact to spend every birthday together doing some kind of challenge. This would be a big birthday for Eilish. She was turning sixty. I had suggested that we do something extra special this year. There was a place I had been with Jim and the kids the year before, where we stayed in a mobile home. It was a beautiful part of Wales, called Pembrokeshire. We decided that's where we would go, and we would walk the coastal trails. This had all been decided before I knew that my cancer was back.

Now that the date was approaching, I was determined to be able to go. I didn't want to let Eilish down and it would also be something of a milestone for me, to be able to make it to Wales for our special birthday trip.

'Are you sure about this?' Eilish asked me as we set off to catch the ferry. 'We can always leave it for another time,' she said, worried that I may not be feeling well enough to go.

'I'm sure,' I said. 'I've been dreaming about this for so long.'

When I had booked the tickets for the ferry, I had looked at the date: October seemed a very long way away. I tried to visualise myself walking along the coast with Eilish. I had kept that image with me, as the date got ever closer.

Now, here we were, setting off for Wales, just as we planned. I couldn't believe it. We were giddy with the thought as we stepped onto the ferry. After a few hours we docked, rented a car and made our way to Pembrokeshire.

For three days we walked along the golden beaches, looking out at the azure blue ocean. We walked slowly, at our own pace. I could feel the breeze against my skin, and nature surrounding me. I was drinking it in. The world was alive with colour, and I was alive to see it.

We sat on the beach and watched the sun sinking in the west, like an orange ball melting into the water. I closed my eyes for a moment to take it all in. When I opened them I was crying. Eilish and I looked at one another. She was crying too. 'Happy birthday!' we said, almost in unison. We laughed and gave one another a hug. Unspoken, but we both knew the significance of that moment – we had survived another lap around the sun, another year on earth. We were walking on sacred ground – the space between life and death. And it was beautiful.

We returned to Ireland, revitalised. Ready to take on the world again.

45

Pembro

I TURNED ON MY COMPUTER. A notification from
Facebook popped up. There were fourteen new friend
requests. I scrolled through the list of names, examining their
profile photos. There were no names or faces I recognised. This
happened nearly every day now, new requests from people I
had never met. My inbox was full of messages from strangers –
women and men from across the country desperate for answers.
They were racing against the clock. Or their wives or husbands
were, or their sisters or brothers or mums or dads. The messages
were heart-breaking, each one struggling with the ultimate
question of life and death. They had explored all avenues, been
through chemotherapy and radiotherapy. Nothing had worked.
They were coming to me to ask for advice about clinical trials
and drugs and therapies. I took a deep breath. How had I
become the authority on cancer? I closed the laptop.

That night as I lay in bed, the messages kept running through
my mind.

'My dad was diagnosed ...'

'My sister is just thirty-five years old ...'

'I'm a mum of three children ...'

All those people out there, with families and people they love, struggling to cling to life.

I remembered how much it meant to me when people responded to my posts on the forum when I had post-natal depression, how much I needed that at the time, how much of a lifeline it was.

The next morning I opened my laptop to check my email. The red icon on the Facebook screen showed more requests, more messages. I started on the first one on the list and decided I would try to write back to five people a day, working through their questions one at a time.

I worked out a schedule so that I would have enough time to research the problem in each message and the clinical trials available. I gathered together the best information I could find but every time I wrote back to someone I was careful to remind them that I was not an expert. I've always been good at research; I knew how to manoeuvre through the websites, documents and technical lingo. I speedily read long reviews of the trials and personal testimonies, trying to string it all together, to find out what seemed to be working and what wasn't, searching through the data in the worldwide quest for a cure for cancer.

Sometimes I cannot believe there is still an illness we cannot cure. I know one day, and it may be someday very soon, they will have a cure. I'm sure we will look back at chemotherapy – hooking people up to intravenous infusions, filling them with chemicals – and wonder how we ever allowed that to happen.

There is something terribly amiss, I thought, when people around the country can't access information from their doctors and feel their only option is to reach out to me. I put a reminder in my notepad to look into what kinds of systems existed that could help people access information. It seemed bizarre that their doctors and consultants wouldn't provide this information. But I knew from my own experience that this was the case.

The consultants tell you their plan of action. They tell you exactly what the options are. Only that there aren't any options. They use words like 'palliative' – words that mean no hope. How can that be the only way?

I could feel the anger rising in me, with every desperate message I read. People deserved better.

There was something inherently wrong about what was happening. There had been an acknowledgement that we had been let down by the state, and we were being given access to Pembro, which seemed to be working for some. But there were hundreds of other women in Ireland, outside of the 221+ group, who were also suffering from cervical cancer and they still didn't have the option of trying this drug as it was still unlicensed for cervical cancer in Ireland. It had only been sanctioned for those affected by the scandal.

Labour TD Alan Kelly had been in touch about doing something to highlight this. He suggested that I, along with one of the women who was trying to get access to Pembro, could go on the *Claire Byrne Live* show. Someone came to mind immediately; her name was Áine Morgan. I had met her at a talk I gave in Galway. She'd come up to me after and told me that she had Stage 4 cervical cancer and was running out of options. We swapped numbers and kept in touch. I told Alan that I would talk to Áine about doing the show.

Something more had to be done. We made a plan and issued a statement about the need for women who had cervical cancer who were not included in the 221+ group to have access to Pembro. Both Áine and I appeared on *Claire Byrne Live* on RTÉ television to speak on the issue.

As I sat on the panel, I looked around me and took in what was happening. I thought about the sheer injustice of the situation. To my left was TD Alan Kelly and Áine. Áine was just like me: she was a young woman, she had a life, she had been given a terminal diagnosis. But the difference between us was that I was receiving Pembro and she wasn't. I was getting a chance to fight for life, and she wasn't.

On my right was the man in charge of pharmaceutical licensing in Ireland, Professor Michael Barry, representing the National Centre for Pharmacoeconomics (NCPE), the body that decides whether people like me and Áine are given access to these medicines. Pembro was only licensed in Ireland for three types of cancer – non small-cell lung cancer, Hodgkin lymphoma and melanoma.

As the conversation progressed I was reminded of the court case. It all came down to money. Human lives, what are they worth? My life. Áine's life. To us and the people we love, they were worth everything. So many things in the world come down to cost – the economics of lives. Were we worth the cost of this drug? Could the government justify the spend?

But what was the cost of us not surviving? There would be children without mothers, husbands without wives, mothers without daughters.

Áine spoke of her desperation. She didn't have long to live. She was trying to fundraise enough money to pay for Pembro –

the thousands it would cost for each infusion. Her friends and family were rallying round, but time was running out.

The debate continued as Claire Byrne diligently chaired the panel, challenging each participant and getting to the heart of the matter. As we sat side by side in that studio, the reality was stark. Could the state put more value on the life of one citizen over another? It was clear this couldn't go on.

Our appearance on the show would have an impact. I had texted Simon Harris just before I went on to give him the heads-up that he would probably have a bit of firefighting on his hands the following day. I didn't apologise for what I was about to say. Simon knew me well enough at this point to know that I do these things to help other people and because it is the right thing to do. He took it on the chin but the appearance did put him under a huge amount of pressure. The NCPE were very clear about their position: Pembro is not licensed for cervical cancer and the minister must remember this. There was a bit of a backlash on Twitter from some media and patient representatives for other cancers who wanted the drug licensed for their cancer too. I felt guilty, but I hoped that it might pave the way for people with other cancers to also gain access to new drugs eventually.

Alan Kelly and I kept in touch after the *Claire Byrne Live* appearance. We waited to see if an announcement would come, but there was nothing. Alan feared that the minister was being put under pressure. He suggested a presentation in the Dáil audio-visual room to politicians from all parties, believing that cross-party support was essential if we were to get this over the line. He also said that we needed another woman, like Áine, to appear and tell her story.

I had just the woman in mind – Tracey Brennan. Tracey and I

had met over the summer. Tracey, like Áine, had Stage 4 cervical cancer and was doing alright on the palliative chemotherapy, but she wanted to keep her options open and have Pembro as a backup for when she finished her current palliative chemotherapy course. We met at St Vincent's Hospital one day in July. Tracey drove all the way from Roscommon to meet me. She was still bald from the chemotherapy; her hair was only starting to grow back. She was bubbly, full of positivity and great craic. We talked so much that day that I realised I had missed my train to Galway, where I was giving a talk that evening. Tracey, without blinking, offered to drive me there and then drive herself back to Roscommon. I tried to argue but it was pointless. Anyway, it gave us more time to chat and I just about made my talk in Galway on time.

I called Tracey to propose coming to speak with us in the Dáil. She was up for it. And so, Áine, Tracey and I, along with our oncologist, Dr David Fennelly, appeared before the TDs in the Dáil AV room to present the case for prescribing Pembro. Dr Fennelly backed up our stories with his professional medical opinion and we left feeling that we had won the politicians over.

Alan Kelly took us to the Dáil bar to have a celebratory drink and we observed the voting that was taking place in the chamber, which went on until well after midnight that night. It was the night the Dáil passed the landmark bill providing for access to abortion. We were there when the bill was passed – another milestone for the women of Ireland. We clinked our glasses in celebration. What a night to be present in Leinster House.

A few weeks later the government announced they would be granting access to Pembro to all the women affected with cervical cancer on a case-by-case basis in public hospitals when a treating clinician determines that this is in the patient's best interests. When I heard the news I was overjoyed. I knew what this meant. I knew what it was like to sit on a recliner chair, barely able to move, while your cancer grew. I knew what it was like to be without any options, thinking you were going to die. I knew the difference Pembro had made to my life – it had given me my life back, if even just for a time. At least now the other women, women like Áine and Tracey, would also stand a chance.

We were conscious of the need to keep joy in the children's lives. With everything going on around them, it was important to keep a sense of normality, to keep the fun alive. As November crept into December, we bought Christmas jumpers and Santa hats. We decided to get festive early in December, to make the most of the Christmas spirit. It was the children's favourite time of year and we wanted it to be a happy time for them. They deserved a break.

We decided to get a dog, something to cheer the kids up. They had wanted one for years. We had imagined getting something small and fluffy, as we didn't have a large house. The kids had other plans, however. They chose a big black and white bulldog and named him Alfie, who would soon become the centre of our home.

I was invited to turn on the Christmas lights in Limerick. We put on our winter coats, bundled into the car and headed for the city centre. There was a towering Christmas tree, with colourful decorations and a festive atmosphere about the town. The crowds gathered in the square. Christmas music was playing loudly as people sang along to Christmas carols. And then the big moment came. I was called to the stage. I looked out at Limerick city – the place I had come to call home. Amelia and Darragh stood with me as the crowd counted us down: Three ... two ... one! We pressed the button and the Christmas lights lit up the town. The crowds cheered. It was officially Christmas in Limerick.

For me it was especially poignant because I didn't think I'd live to see another Christmas. I watched the lights twinkling. Darragh pointed at the star at the top of the tree. I put my arms around the children and held them close. This was happiness.

46

What A Difference A Year Makes

I WOKE EARLY THAT DAY. I could see the light of the morning sun making its way through the parting in the curtains. It felt like spring, even though it was still January, 12 January to be exact. I knew that date well. It was ingrained in my memory.

It was my anniversary. Exactly twelve months since I sat opposite the doctor who told me I had twelve months to live. I had survived the year. And what a year it had been.

The day ahead was going to be a difficult one. It was someone else's anniversary too. There was a mass being held for a woman I had never met, but who'd had a huge impact on my life. Her name was Emma. She had died exactly one year ago. She was the very same age as me when she died of cervical cancer, leaving behind her husband and three young daughters.

She was the wife of Peter, the man who had emailed me after *The Ray D'Arcy Show*, who had helped me to try to get onto the clinical trial in America and who gave me hope that it was possible for me to get on Pembro. I owed everything to him.

The anniversary mass was held in the church in Rathgar in Dublin. Peter was outside greeting people when I arrived. I felt very emotional as I approached. I tried to hold it together when I was talking to him. I told him the only reason I was still alive was because of the drug, and it was because of his email that I had tried so hard to get access to it. I explained how I felt I owed him so much. He said he felt he owed a great deal to me.

He gestured towards his three daughters, Jessica, Catherine and Amelia. 'I never want this to happen to them.'

I gave him a hug and entered the church for the service. How thin, I thought, the veil between life and death. As the organ played, in the quiet privacy of the pew, I began to cry.

All I kept thinking was: Please, don't let me die. Not yet. Not yet.

I was becoming very tired again. The constant media interviews and meetings were taking a lot out of me, but I needed to keep going. We needed answers and systemic change: proof that this could never happen again.

'You need to take a break, Vicky.' I was hearing it from everyone in my family. They didn't understand how important this campaign was in keeping me alive. If I stopped, I was scared I would fall over. That would be that. So I kept going. But then I fell anyway.

I had been feeling particularly unwell for two or three days. I was running high temperatures and vomiting a lot. I was due to go to St Vincent's Hospital for treatment that week so I decided to wait until I was in the hospital to broach these new symptoms with the oncology team.

The day of the appointment, I decided to drive up to Dublin, instead of taking the train. I was test driving a new car, a Volvo, and I felt fine when I started off that morning. Stephen had been talking to me about buying a Volvo ever since he had met me, so I had decided to try one out. Instead of putting off the test drive, me being me, of course I went ahead with it. It was a bad idea. Although I felt fine when I started off that morning, I was an hour into the drive when I could feel my temperature rising. I was starting to sweat. I rolled down the window to breathe some fresh air, hoping that would help. I started shivering and was alternating between feeling hot and cold. I tried to concentrate on the road, but my head was starting to pound. The headache was getting worse and worse.

I pulled into a service station to take some paracetamol to try to bring my temperature down. I rang the oncology ward to let them know I was feeling unwell and that I would be late. Somehow, I managed to get back on the road, and make it to the hospital.

I walked into the ward, feeling weak, like I was in a daze. Lisa, one of the administrative team, took one look at me and got me to a bed.

As I lay there I wondered if this was it, how it would end. The ward was noisy. The phone continued to ring – journalists looking for interviews, people from the campaign getting in touch. Things were always moving. I didn't have the energy to answer the calls. I was nauseous all the time, coupled with the guilt of not getting back to people. I decided I needed to take some time to myself. The only way to do it would be to announce it publicly, that way the news stations would know not to call for a little while.

I put up a tweet and sent it out. The story ran on the morning news bulletins. The phone stopped ringing. I breathed a sigh of relief. I spent the next week in St Vincent's Hospital in Dublin, before they decided it was safe for me to go home.

When I got home the house seemed quiet. I wasn't running around anywhere, or answering calls. It was the first time I had stopped in a long time. It was strange having time to myself again. I didn't have the energy to go outside, so I pottered around the house. Occasionally, I forced myself to bring Alfie for short walks; it was good for both of us. It kept me moving, kept the blood pumping, and was a chance to get some air.

I had asked people not to contact me, but as soon as they stopped, everything felt deathly quiet, like I was back to being just Vicky again – a mammy, a wife, a daughter. There was something frightening about that. At least when I was on the campaign it became about something else, something bigger than me. I didn't have time to remember I was sick.

Now, I was finding it hard to get out of bed. I was tired all the time and nauseous. I felt like a sick person again. I worried that the infection could be a sign that the Pembro had stopped working or that my body was beginning to act against it.

I could hear the voice of the consultant, just over twelve months ago, telling me that I had only a year to live. How did they know? I had done everything in my power to keep going, to defy the odds. To prove them wrong. And yet, it seemed the horse was chasing once again, getting closer and closer.

At the dinner table I noticed Amelia's nails. They were chewed and torn. How had I not noticed this before, I wondered. I looked over at her. She was biting her lip and I could see she was agitated. She must have been doing it a lot. A sign she was feeling anxious.

That night when Darragh had gone to bed I asked Amelia if she fancied a cup of tea. She offered to bring it up to me in bed.

'No, petto, I'll come down for it.'

I wanted to have a good chat with her. We started talking about school and how that was going. Good, she said. And she was getting on very well with her friends.

'Mam, I want to give up lifesaving.'

Here it was, I knew there was something. 'Oh, why? I thought you were enjoying that.'

She explained that in every lesson there was an exercise where someone had to pretend to be drowning and had to be rescued. It was an example to the rest of the class, to watch how it was done. 'I hate everyone looking at me,' she said.

I tried to listen first, before coming out with my opinion. I had been working on that lately, especially with the kids. 'Oh, and what way does that make you feel?' I asked.

She explained that it made her feel anxious to have everyone watching. She looked distressed talking about it.

I could see there was something bigger going on. I explained that lifesaving was a very good thing to know how to do. 'I remember when lifesaving helped me through a very difficult time in my life,' I told her, thinking back to my college year after the accident.

I convinced her to keep it up, to give it a few more weeks and to see how she felt about it then. I also suggested we go and talk to someone about lifesaving and why it was making her feel that way – to see if we could make things better. After a few minutes, she agreed that that would be a good idea.

I wondered how long this had been going on – if I'd been missing the signs while I was busy rushing in and out. This was the top priority now – making sure the kids were okay.

I knew she must be worried about me. I was glad I was there with her, there for her to talk to me, to tell me what was going through her mind. I worry about what life will be like for Amelia when she is older, when things are less innocent. School days can be difficult, but there's also a shelter in that community – of knowing you belong somewhere and having the structure of rules and responsibilities. When you get a bit older, you have to create your own life. I have to be here for that. I need to be here, to be able to help her through that. It would kill me if I wasn't.

I wanted to get five more years, enough to see Amelia turn twenty.

Everything I had done over the past year, everything I had fought for, had been for Amelia. I see incredible strength in her. She has been through so much in her short life already. And yet somehow she still finds some way to bounce back, to come back smiling. Kids are amazing that way. We can learn so much from them.

47

Wishing Well

A S THE WEEKS WENT BY I was starting to get my strength back. The infection had cleared up and life was getting back to normal. I decided to bring Darragh for an outing to Kildare Village to buy shoes and other things for his upcoming birthday trip to Legoland, which he was really looking forward to.

When we were finished shopping, we were walking back out through the courtyard. Darragh tugged on my sleeve. 'Can I have a coin please, Mam?' he asked.

I looked in my purse and found a coin.

'Thanks, Mam!' he said. He walked to the fountain in the middle of the courtyard, tossed the coin into the water and closed his eyes for a few seconds.

I took his hand and we walked towards the car park. 'What did you wish for?' I asked, thinking he would say a football or a rugby ball or something.

'I wished for you to get better, Mammy,' he said.

I squeezed his hand. I loved him so much. He was so young, just eight years old, with a world of worries on his shoulders. And he was minding me already.

48

Daffodils

I T WAS SPRINGTIME AGAIN AND the daffodils were out in bloom. Each one standing proudly in the earth, like a tribute to those who have fallen. Over the following few months, between March and May I watched as two more women I cared deeply about passed away from cervical cancer.

In March I received word that Laura Brennan, who was just twenty-six years old, had died. She had been too old to receive the HPV vaccine when it was rolled out, but she had become an avid campaigner for it. She believed that if she'd received it, she would have lived. Instead, she was trying to come to terms with the fact that she was going to die.

Not long before she passed away, she appeared on *The Late Late Show* with Ryan Tubridy. She spoke about having cancer, and the fear of what was to come, as her health deteriorated: 'Sometime in the future, there might not be a cure for my cancer and I will be in pain, and I won't be able to get out of bed,' she said. 'I know my parents will take good care of me like they always do – I'm so lucky. But they'll come up and ask me am I okay, and I'll be in pain. I know I'll tell them I'm grand, or I'll crack a joke, and they'll give me a smile back. But in their eyes, I'll see pain.'

Her words were powerful, her strength so admirable. Laura worked tirelessly to create awareness about the importance of the HPV vaccine, which aims to prevent this terrible disease.

We had met just once, for a coffee in Ennis. I had been so taken by her strength of spirit, especially at such a young age. We had kept in touch ever since, and I watched with admiration as she worked in the hope of improving the lives of the next generation. In her short life, she'd had an enormous impact. The uptake of the vaccine had increased by twenty per cent in one year, due in no small part to her work.

A few weeks later, Ruth Morrissey, who was also directly affected by the scandal, was back in court, challenging the HSE and the laboratories in the same way I had done a year previously. Despite the promises from the government, no alternative to the High Court route had yet been created for Ruth or any of the other 221 women. Ruth had already been through a long and arduous process, bringing her case to the High Court. It had begun in July 2018 and had been adjourned until 2019. She was still fighting, both her cancer and her case.

I thought of the day I met the taoiseach and I remembered the government's assurances that this would not happen anymore. The government had promised that no other women should have to go through what I and Emma Mhic Mhathúna had gone through – having to fight our cases in the courts, at our most vulnerable. They had promised that cases could be settled by mediation, or by tribunal (which they intended to establish). So far, this hadn't happened.

And so, here she was – a terminally ill woman battling through a major court case. I was in awe of her strength and determination. I was rooting for her every day and watching the trial coverage closely. I met with her one afternoon, a week before the trial ended, to see how she was coping. She seemed confident that they had a strong case. Cian was working with her as her solicitor and they were hopeful of a good outcome. She was in a lot of pain, though, and her health seemed to be deteriorating. I knew what she must be going through. I had sat in that same seat in court. I knew how exhausted she must have been. Ruth had told the court she did not think she would ever have been told about the review of smear tests if it had not been for my case, one year previously. It made me think of what could have happened had I signed that gagging order. Ruth, and so many others, may never have known the truth.

Then one night, we got word that Judge Kevin Cross, who had presided over this case too, would be giving a ruling the following day. Rather than settling, like my case, and others, this one was the first to go to judgement. We waited tentatively to see what would happen. This ruling could have huge implications.

He awarded Ruth and her husband 2.16 million euro in damages. All three defendants were held jointly and equally liable; this meant that all three defendants were equally liable for the damages in Ruth's case, save for an amount of ten thousand euro, which the HSE were forced to pay for the non-disclosure of the audit.

I felt somewhat vindicated. Finally, the HSE were being found to be liable for all aspects of our national cervical screening programme. Up to this point, the HSE had hidden behind the labs, to whom they had sub-contracted out the reading of our smears. Now, Judge Cross had exposed their role and forced them to accept their responsibility in errors resulting from the screening programme, which he had found them ultimately responsible for. Not only that, he went a step further: he ruled, crucially, that labs carrying out screening programmes should have 'absolute confidence' in their decision if they are giving a sample the all-clear.

This would have huge implications for other women taking cases in the future, and for the future of cervical screening. It is still not known what ways this will affect screening in Ireland. Both the HSE and the labs went on to appeal various issues in the judgement. I can only hope that the judgement will not be overturned and that it will pave the way for a safer screening programme that the women of Ireland can trust once again, and that some good will have come of all of this.

Ruth and her husband Paul stood in that same spot outside the court where Jim and I had stood, just one year ago, and addressed the media. She said she now wanted to spend the little time she had left with her daughter Libby.

Less than a week later I got a text from Paul to tell me that Ruth had received bad news. Her cancer had spread and she was in a hospice for pain management.

Later the very same day, I was on my way to the month's mind mass for Laura Brennan when I got a phone call from Stephen to tell me that Tracey Brennan had died. The news floored me. I attended the month's mind for Laura Brennan with the news of Ruth's deteriorating health and Tracey's death in my head. I met Laura's parents and they invited me back to their home. We sat over a cup of tea in their kitchen and talked – about Laura, about life, about cancer. There was something shared in all this – a common knowledge of the strength of love and loss.

Tracey's funeral was heart-breaking. My mind could not comprehend that this had happened to her, that she was gone. I thought back to the day we stood in front of the Dáil, only a few months previously, and made the case for Pembro to be made available to all women with cervical cancer in Ireland. When the news had been announced a few days later that the government was to grant our wishes, Tracey had been overjoyed. She had texted me immediately: *Hey ya Mrs, I have the most fantastic feeling of relief today with the amazing news. Thank you so much for all the support and encouragement. You have so much to be proud of in all the craziness.*

She had been full of plans for her future. We had talked about her applying for a position as a patient advice liaison officer, which she would have been brilliant at. She'd wanted my advice and a bit of coaching for the interview. None of us had thought that Tracey wouldn't make it. I'd been convinced she would make a comeback, once she was receiving Pembro, the way I had done. But for Tracey, it was too little, too late. She had only had two infusions of Pembro before cancer took her from this world. She was only thirty-three. She left behind her husband Aidan and three-year-old son Evan.

I went to Tracey's funeral even though I'd rather have been anywhere else. It was absolutely heart-breaking. I saw Evan being taken in and out of the church during the funeral mass to go to the toilet, or to get sweets. He was smiling, unaware of what was going on around him. I met Tracey's husband Aidan, who was utterly bereft. They had been together since they were teenagers. I met her mam, Pauline, who looked barely older than me – she is only fifty-two – and I met Tracey's sisters. Amanda, one of her sisters, was due to have a baby the week after the funeral. They told me that Tracey had been trying to hold on for the baby.

I went to visit Ruth in the hospice that same week. It was a strange mixture of emotions. I congratulated her on the result of the trial. I told her how much the ruling in her case would matter, what a difference it would make for the women of Ireland. She smiled. But there was a sadness none of us spoke of, to see her lying in her hospice bed. She was in great form, putting on a brave face, and talking and joking, the way people do, somehow, even at this most difficult time. Because it's all you can do. But I am sure she could see the pain in my eyes. Neither Ruth nor I were under any illusion that, as with me, it was only a matter of time now.

I spent the following week trying to recover from all the loss, trying to understand why life can be so bloody cruel, trying not to become bitter, trying not to panic about my own situation. I tried not to go to that place that I sometimes go to and start planning my funeral and picturing myself dead. I knew that if I started this, I would have given up, somehow. I tried to focus on life and living. That was what Tracey wanted. That is what we all want, ultimately, to really live and enjoy life.

And so, I pulled myself together and the following weekend I went home to Mooncoin and walked in the Midnight Walk, which I was unable to do twelve months previously when the walk was organised to raise funds for me.

By the light of the moon shining down on the place that was once my home, where I learned to walk as a baby, where I learned to walk as a teenager after the car accident, I put one foot in front of the other and walked in honour of Tracey and Laura and Emma Mhic Mhathúna and Emma Kearns and Julie and Irene and Alice and Orla, and all the other women who had died from this horrible cancer, and I vowed to continue living, to keep up the fight, for as long as I could.

My brother Lee and his partner Diane had asked me to be godmother to their baby months before their baby was born. It was a wonderful surprise. I was already godmother to my nephew, Tyler and my niece, Phoebe. I wasn't expecting to be asked a third time.

'We're going to name her Daisy,' he told me. 'Daisy Victoria, after you.'

I hugged him. My eyes were welling up with tears. 'I'm honoured,' I said.

He looked at me for a moment. I knew what he was saying, and not saying. He wanted me to be there, to stand for her on her christening day. He was trying to give me something to aim for, something to live for.

Well, just a few weeks ago, I held little Daisy Victoria in my arms at her christening. I have fallen in love with my new goddaughter, who is the most placid, happy baby. As I held Daisy, I looked around at all the family and friends who had gathered in the church … for a christening instead of the funeral I had imagined, my own funeral. I thought how wonderful life is, even when everything is thrown at you. It is what you do with it and who you spend it with that matters and I was spending it with the people who matter most to me. And I hoped that Daisy Victoria would grow up accepting that life is difficult, but it is worth living and celebrating, every day, right to the end.

49

Whispers On A Sea Breeze

I HAVE ALWAYS BEEN DRAWN to water. My father was a fisherman, and his father before him. Maybe it is in my blood. They say the human body is made up almost entirely of water. There must be something familiar about it for us, as a species. It feels like home.

I come to the ocean whenever I need to think. Or not think. Lately it's about not thinking. Just being. Watching the constant ebb and flow of the water along the shore. There's something very dependable about it. Very reassuring. What goes out must come back in. The intake of breath by the sea, as the tide goes out, and the relief when it returns again, water covering the sand once more, then pulling the pebbles and shells back with it. Breaths. Each one is sacred. Though we spend most of our lives not thinking about it. Breathing.

There is a story I once heard about a little wave who was making his way across the sea. He was getting closer and closer to the shore and he began to be afraid. He was scared about what would happen when he crashed into the shore. One of the older waves took him aside and asked him why he was worried. I don't know what will happen to me when it happens, he told the older wave. The older wave turned to him and said, 'Well, look at me. You needn't be afraid. Because one day you will crash into the shore. You will no longer be the little wave, but you will become part of the sea once more.'

I want my ashes to be spread here when I die. Whenever that day may come. To make one final journey along this beach. To become part of the sea once more.

We all have a beginning and an end.

Whatever happens next, I know that my struggles will not have been in vain. Everything that happened in my life, happened to make me, me. And in the end, I hope that my life will have meant something. It will have been worth something.

I still think about death sometimes. I'm not afraid of it anymore. I know it will happen. I just don't know when. The hardest part for me, it's not the dying, it's leaving my children behind. That's what breaks my heart.

I think of the kind of woman Amelia will become. And I hope that the world will be a better place for her, because of what we, the women of Ireland, have been through and what we have stood for.

I think of Darragh's coin shimmering in the light, at the bottom of the fountain. His wish for me. I close my eyes and make a wish for him, and for Amelia.

I wish that one day they will hear my story, so that they will know who their mother was and why she did the things she did; that they'll read this book and they will understand me. But more than that, that it will be a source of courage for them, no matter what they face in life. If I am not there to face the darkness with them, I hope that they will know in their hearts that I am standing with them. They will see from my story that, no matter what happens in life, no matter what is thrown at them, they have the strength to stand up to it, to get up and face another day, and to do what they believe is right, no matter how hard that might be.

My wish is that they too will find the strength to overcome. And to know that I am right there with them, every step of the way.

Because we all have that strength in us, the strength to fight for what is right in the world.

My dying wish will be for the women of Ireland – that because of what has happened in this past year, maybe my last year on earth, they will be able to trust that their lives are in safe hands, that they will be minded and cared for at their most vulnerable, and that everything will be done to give them the lives they deserve, the time they deserve, with the people they love and who love them, and who need them in the world.

There will be others who will continue this fight without me, when I'm gone, because we are all in this together, at the end of the day. We all come from that same place – from a mother's womb. This is everybody's story.

I look back at my footprints in the sand. Tomorrow the sea will have washed them away. Ready for new footprints to take their place, to make their mark in the sand. I think of my promise to Amelia that night. A promise I keep every day. To be here as long as I can.

Though recently I feel that black horse chasing me again, getting ever closer. I can hear the clip-clop of his hooves, the tick-tock of the clock as each sacred day passes by. Every sunrise, every sunset, every blessed day. They all count. Every one.

And I know that the day will come that is my last day. My last sunrise, my last sunset.

And then I will be at peace. My ashes will be scattered in the water, on the silver sands of the beach at Doughmore.

And I will become part of the sea once more.

Part of the wild Atlantic Ocean ... where only the white horses can catch me.

Vicky Phelan Acknowledgements

There are so many people who have helped to make this book a reality, from those who assisted in the writing and editing process, to those who reminded me of stories that have gone in to the book, to my family, friends, colleagues and unnamed individuals who have helped me, in whatever way, to get me to where I am today, alive and kicking and going nowhere!

To my ghost-writer, Naomi Linehan, I simply could not have done this without you. You brought life to my story on the page in a way that I did not think was possible. Towards the end, I felt like if I simply had a thought, that you would know it before I expressed it, such was your amazing ability to get into my head. Thank you, quite simply, does not cover it.

To the wonderful team at Hachette Ireland – to Breda Purdue and Ciara Considine for taking a chance on me and allowing me to tell my story. To Elaine Egan and Joanna Smyth for navigating me through the PR and marketing stuff around the release of this book, and for facilitating me with all my commitments. To Aonghus Meaney for his copy-editing. Thank you one and all.

To my agent Sheila Crowley for believing that my story was worth telling and for navigating me through the minefield of getting a book to print.

To my solicitors, Cian O'Carroll and Siobhan Ryan. Thank you for reading through various drafts of this book and for your meticulous attention to detail. You believed in me. You empathised with me. You vindicated me. I cannot thank you enough.

To all the wonderful medical professionals and complementary therapy practitioners whom I have dealt with over the years, some of whom are mentioned in this book. Thank you for your compassion, empathy and patient-centred care.

To Stephen Teap and Lorraine Walsh, two people whom I would never have met had the CervicalCheck debacle not been exposed following my court case. I am so glad that our paths have crossed, regardless of the awful circumstances. Thank you for your unwavering support over the past year and for listening to me going on about the book.

To my wonderful, wonderful friends of which I have many. Some who are mentioned in the book, many others who are not.

To my best friends Maria and Susan. I simply would not be me without you!

To the Mooncoin gang – Patrick, Peter, Bernard, Paul, Laura, Sean, Siobhan, Sinead. Thanks for keeping me grounded.

To the Carrigeen girlies – Lucy, Siobhan, Anita, Maeve and Ana. Thanks for either minding my kids, having a bottle of wine and an open door, or making dinners when I was sick.

To my college friends and my UL friends, there are far too many to mention but you know who you are. Thank you for the laughs, the tears, but most importantly the journey.

To Katy, *notre amitié est très important pour moi. Merci de ta patience ces dernières années.*

To the wonderful women of the Literacy Development Centre (LDC) at Waterford Institute of Technology (WIT) where I worked for almost twelve years. To Eilish, Geraldine, Helen, Maeve, Ann-Marie, Therese, Karen, Catherine, Suzanne, Perpetual and Orna – you all kept me on the straight and narrow over the years when I struggled either with overcoming depression or with one of the many events that happened to me during my time working with you, from Amelia's terrible accident to my cancer, to finding out that my cancer was back. I owe you my sanity. Without your constant support and many shoulders to cry on, I simply would not have been able to carry on at times.

To my 'Mammy' friends – women whom I have made friends with as a result of having children the same age. I would be lost without all of you! Thank you for keeping me sane, for taking my children off my hands and giving me a bit of 'me' time – and for rowing in and being there when I got sick.

To my aunts Ann and Tina, who were my safe haven when I stayed down for my three working days at WIT. You helped me more than you will ever know.

To all those whose lives have touched mine, even if only briefly, and who I mention in the book, from those whose simple kindness brought me back from the brink to those who helped to shape the person I am today. I cannot possibly thank everyone individually here. I would rather thank you privately.

To my family. To Mam and Dad, I hope that I have done you proud. I love you so much it hurts. There are not enough ways to thank you both for all the sacrifices that you have made for me over the years. For all of the hardship that my life has brought to your door (and there has been a lot!), I honestly do not know how you are both still standing, but it is you who have taught me resilience and to stand up again and to keep living. Thank you.

To my sister, Lyndsey – as anyone who knows us both will tell you, we are like chalk and cheese. If you didn't know, you would never think that we were related, so different are we! Lyndsey is the fun, glamorous one while I am the serious, studious (and generally more sensible!) one. Thank you for always being there for me, even when you didn't know it. I worry less for Amelia when I am gone with you in her life.

To my three brothers – Robbie, Lee and Jonnie. Thank you for toughening me up. I had to learn to fight my corner as the oldest with three boys coming behind me. It has served me well in life. Thank you also for being wonderful uncles to Amelia and Darragh.

To Jim – thank you for supporting me throughout the process of writing this book which, I know, has not been easy for you. Thank you for staying the course through all that has been thrown at us. Thank you for always allowing me to be me, even when that has been difficult for you, and, most importantly, thank you for the gift of Amelia and Darragh in our lives.

To Amelia and Darragh – thank you for giving me two wonderful reasons to live every day. I love you more than you will ever know and I always will.

Naomi Linehan Acknowledgements

A most heartfelt thanks goes to Vicky, for telling your story – for everything you have been through and continue to go through and for the hope and strength you give to others. It has been the greatest honour working so closely with you. To Ciara Considine for her unwavering guidance and support and to everyone at Hachette for making this book possible. Special thanks to Cian O'Carroll and his team. And to all the people who contributed in so many ways to tell this powerful story.

This book was written while travelling the waterways of Ireland by barge with my wonderful husband Ben, who spent manys a day at the tiller so that I could be at the proverbial typewriter! To Ben, for being the incredible person you are, every day to everyone, for your constant love and support and for all the adventures past and to come. To 'Plum' the baby we are so excited to meet in a few months' time. To my mother, Teresa, and sister, Laura, who are and always have been my world, always so close to my heart. To Dallan, the brother I always hoped for. To all the Linehans and Dillons and Kitchins – every one of whom I adore and am blessed to have as part of my family. And to all the friends in life who make the world the wonderful place that it is. You have all been such an amazing support on this journey.

A very special mention goes to my dad, Shay, who passed away during the publication of this book after a brave battle with cancer. He was and always will be my guiding light in life – the most loving, inspirational father, best friend, and gifted writer. For all the love and magic you brought into the world. Loved with all our hearts, and missed every day.

This one's for you, Dad.